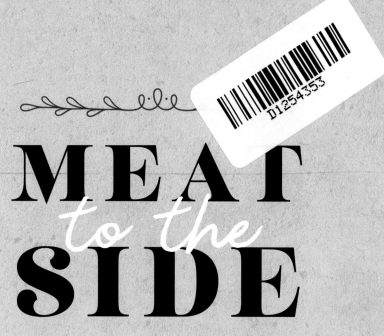

MEAT
to the
SIDE

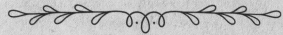

A **PLANT-FORWARD** Guide to
Bringing **BALANCE** to Your Plate

LIREN BAKER

VICTORY BELT PUBLISHING
LAS VEGAS

First published in 2021 by Victory Belt Publishing, Inc.

ISBN-13: 978-1-628604-44-3

Cover design by Kat Lannom

Front and back cover photos by Tatiana Briceag

Interior design by Crizalie Olimpo and Charisse Reyes

Interior photos by Liren Baker

Illustrations by Eli San Juan

Printed in Canada
TC 0121

For Thomas, who led us down our
plant-forward path, and for
Caeli and Carsten for
eating their vegetables

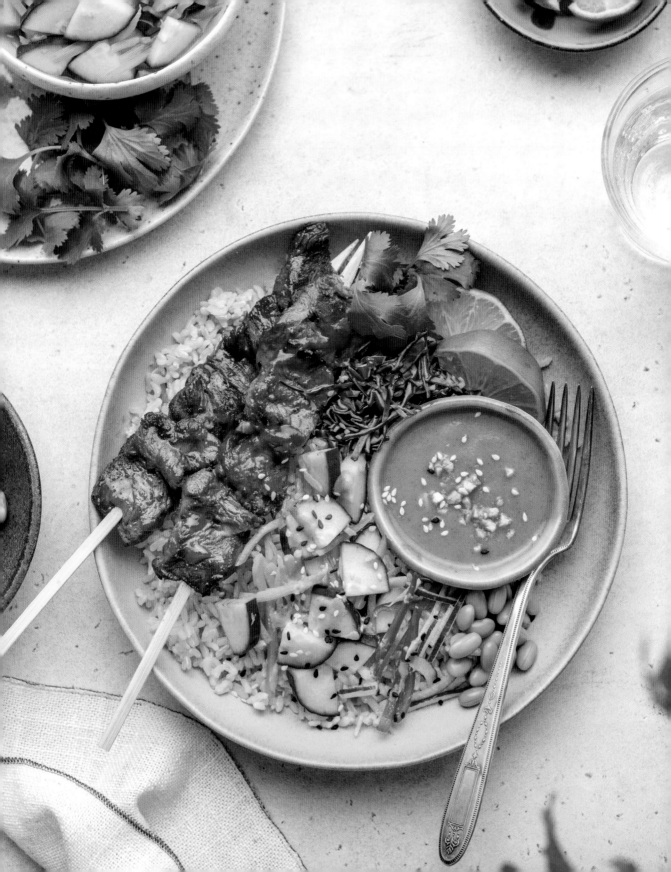

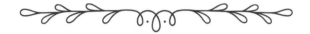

CONTENTS

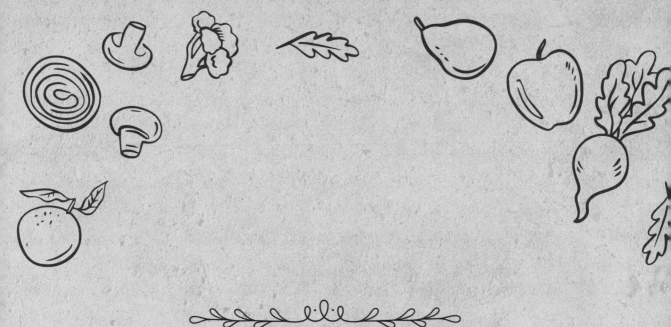

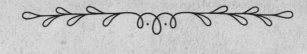

INTRODUCTION

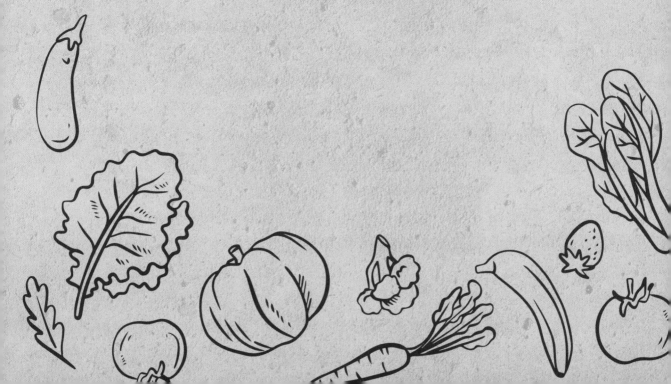

Let's cut to the chase. I don't like the word *diet.* For too many people, *diet* is used to describe restrictive eating, with a focus on regulation and weight loss. To me, eating is about celebrating, nourishing, and fueling our bodies so they perform at their best.

But, like many people, I've taken my own food journey that has led me to dabble in different ways of cooking and eating. I grew up an omnivore, eating pretty much anything. Nothing was off the table at my house—my mother grew incredible vegetables, and our garden was lush with all kinds of produce in the summer. Our freezer was full of fish that my uncle caught off the Long Island Sound. I loved growing up in New York and traveling around the globe as a family, exposed to a melting pot of flavors that primed my palate to enjoy all kinds of foods.

Those who know me know that I will eat just about anything; there are very few foods I won't ever taste or try. So the idea of omitting something from my diet was tough for me. That said, as I got older and had a family of my own, we continued to experiment with food. My daughter suggested we eat pescatarian for one month, and that led to an evolution of our eating habits. We've gone pescatarian, vegan, flexitarian—finally landing on what makes sense for us. If I had to describe how we eat now, it's plant-forward; we still eat meat, but we try our best to place the spotlight on veggies most of the time!

So, rather than omitting meat, this book is about moving it to the side of the plate. It's about finding an achievable balance to nourish and fuel our bodies for a lifetime. It's about finding new ways to add more vegetables to our meals, even in small ways, and reframing how we cook.

I hope you enjoy the recipes in this book and that they inspire you to celebrate the veggies on your plate. Happy cooking!

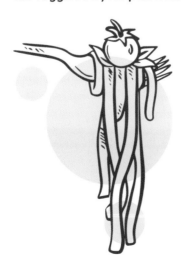

How to Eat More Veggies

Everyone has a unique relationship with vegetables. Perhaps you grew up with parents who were avid gardeners, and picking the fruits and veggies from your backyard inspired a love for fresh produce. Or perhaps you grew up in a city, and your relationship with vegetables was born in the produce aisle at the supermarket. It could be that you grew up on canned and frozen vegetables. Or maybe you visited the farmers market every Saturday. Beyond access, your feelings could depend on taste. Some of us grow up loving the taste of vegetables, while others hate them!

Whatever your relationship with vegetables, I'm guessing you are looking to enhance it (hence this cookbook). While I know some people might simply say, "Eat more veggies!" it's never that simple.

What I do know is that even if you are a die-hard carnivore, there are ways to eat more vegetables. It's all about finding out what works for your lifestyle and your taste buds. That could mean embracing the convenience of frozen vegetables or visiting the farmers market for inspiration. Here are some ways to find vegetable inspiration:

- **Shop the perimeter.** When I'm at the grocery store, I like to start in the produce aisles. That way, my meals are influenced by what is in season. From there, I work my way around the perimeter of the store, where the meat, dairy, and bakery sections are. It's easier to cook fresh meals when your ingredients are fresh and you buy fewer packaged foods, which are shelved in the center of the store. This strategy works especially well if you're like me and look for inspiration when grocery shopping.

- **Visit the farmers market.** It's not always convenient, but what I love about the farmers market is that you are buying your produce directly from the farmers who grew it. They know their food best and are a wonderful source of inspiration. Best of all, you know that you are eating vegetables that are in season locally. Feel free to ask vendors to guide you to vegetables you've never tried, or even ask if they have recipe recommendations!

- **Stock the pantry.** Occasionally, there's nothing fresh left in the fridge—it happens to all of us. For those times, keep a well-stocked pantry. I wholeheartedly embrace canned and frozen vegetables (see page 16 for more on why I think of the freezer and fridge as extensions of the pantry) and often turn to these basics for a delicious veggie-forward meal.

- **Start a garden.** Or maybe just plant your favorite vegetables! Growing your own food is not only rewarding, but it will inspire you to cook the food that you grow. It tastes better, too! I don't mean that you need to have a big vegetable garden—start small. Maybe just plant tomatoes or fresh herbs by the kitchen window at first. Small changes can make a big difference in your eating habits.

But what do you do when you've got all these vegetables in your house? It's time to eat them! You might be surprised to find there are so many ways to incorporate vegetables into every meal.

- **Keep a plate of vegetables and fruit out for snacking.** Just as I am a moth to a flame when I see a charcuterie board, I find that if I prep some vegetables and fruit in the morning and leave them out on the counter, my family is more apt to graze on them throughout the day. It could be as simple as carrots and celery sticks, cherry tomatoes, and mixed berries. I just know that when they're prepped and accessible, they'll be gone by the end of the day!

- **Blitz them in a smoothie.** Smoothies are a daily occurrence for my family; they're the perfect way to sneak in a few extra veggies. I love adding spinach or kale to our smoothies. You can also add avocado, beets, carrots or carrot juice, celery, cucumber, and so much more. Throw some veggies into the blender with some almond milk, along with frozen fruit and a ripe banana for sweetness, and you'll find that drinking your veggies is easy and delicious!

- **Spiralize them.** Don't have a tool like a spiralizer? Not to worry! These days, it's easy to find prespiralized veggies at the grocery store. Zoodles and sweet potato noodles are delicious pasta alternatives. Look for them in the produce or frozen food aisles.

- **Make soup.** If I had to pick just one thing to eat every day of my life, it might be soup. Why? Not only is soup comforting, but it's also one of the easiest ways to add nutrients to a meal. Take chicken noodle soup, for example. Everyone loves a good chicken noodle soup, but why limit it to carrots and celery? Go through your vegetable drawer and add chopped zucchini, spinach, or corn! It's easy to load up the soup and clean out the veggie bin at the same time.

- **Experiment.** Sometimes we make decisions about a vegetable after one bite, when really, all foods deserve a second chance. Peas, for example. Growing up, I was never a fan of the over-boiled peas my mother would serve, but it wasn't until many years later that I experimented with other ways of cooking peas—for example, in a puree, in a simple salad, or as a bright topping for ricotta pizza. I learned to love the little nuggets! So give peas (and other veggies) a chance and try cooking them in various ways. You may be surprised.

- **Add one extra veggie to a dish.** When in doubt, start small. A dish doesn't have to be completely vegetarian. Try adding just one new veggie to every meal, and you will, over the long term, eat more vegetables. To me, that is the bigger gain. It could mean adding a few handfuls of spinach to your soup, some frozen corn to your burrito, or some broccoli to your stir-fry. It all adds up!

Enjoying vegetables is not rocket science—you just have to make it delicious! I would argue that good-quality vegetables harvested at the right time and enjoyed in season don't need much added to them to taste great. But sometimes you don't have access to farm-fresh produce bursting with flavor, or maybe you need a little encouragement to make it appetizing. For that, it's all about flavor.

Flavor can come in many forms, and in this book I discuss ways to add flavor to dishes. But flavor can also come from the proteins you serve with your vegetables. A touch of bacon or pancetta does wonders when you serve it with Brussels sprouts, for example. It's all about rethinking protein and seeing it as a source of flavor so that vegetables can shine.

Rethinking Protein

For me, the key to rethinking protein was finding the right proportions and shifting my focus when eating. During my cooking journey, I realized that perhaps I began to rethink protein when I was a little girl.

When the little version of me would sit at the dinner table and build my plate, I would pile it with the vegetables, rice, and just a *few* pieces of whatever protein was being served. While everyone else might have eaten a larger portion of meat with the veggies as accompaniments, I operated in reverse.

In essence, I was already eating with meat to the side.

I still eat this way today. To me, the meat is flavor, but I prefer to allow the vegetables to be the star of the dish. I know this runs counter to what we see in restaurants, how many people eat at home, and especially how dishes and menus are traditionally built.

I love to adapt old favorites by simply reversing the proportions. Let's take a traditional chicken pot pie as an example. By simply changing the proportions so there are more vegetables in the filling, you can enjoy pot pie with the meat to the side! Another way to approach this is by using less meat and replacing it with a plant protein.

Watch any food show, whether it is a competition or a cooking segment, and the chefs always address a piece of meat or fish as "the protein." However, we often forget that protein can be found in so many foods beyond the butcher counter! Foods like quinoa, lentils, nuts and seeds, beans, soy, and vegetables such as broccoli, spinach, and sweet potatoes are all excellent sources of protein. Once you think beyond meat, you can worry less and enjoy plant-forward eating more.

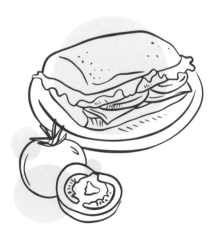

Meaty Substitutes

When embarking on a plant-forward diet, it's common to approach it by looking for meaty substitutes. Many people begin with the good old hamburger. While there are lots of wonderful veggie burgers out there, there are also so many meat substitutes that replicate the juicy, meaty experience of a beef burger. I get it, and occasionally, I will indulge in one of these meaty substitutes myself.

But I've also come to realize that some of these prepackaged solutions are highly processed and, like any indulgence, not something I can eat all the time. Instead, I try to find meaty substitutes among foods that I can easily prepare at home.

Tofu

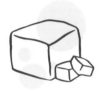

A love for tofu may seem requisite for a plant-based diet, and frankly, soy products sometimes scare people who have never eaten them. I'm here to assure you that you don't need to love tofu to eat plant-forward, but you also have nothing to fear. You just have to learn how to cook it.

The good news is that tofu is delicious, and because it comes in so many forms, it is extremely versatile!

Firm or extra-firm tofu is what most people think of when it comes to replacing meat. Because of its firm texture, it makes a wonderful stand-in for animal protein in many dishes. It works well in place of chicken in a stir-fry noodle dish, for example, because it holds up well to frying and sautéing. You can batter and encrust, deep-fry, and even bake tofu. Since tofu doesn't have its own distinct flavor, it takes on the flavor of any dish extremely well.

Don't forget about other forms of tofu! Medium-firm tofu also works well for frying and baking, though it is a little softer. I love using silken tofu, which is more delicate and custardlike, in everything from desserts like puddings to replacing the eggs in shakshuka.

Mushrooms

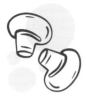

Mushrooms are my favorite meat substitute; you'll find that I build a lot of dishes around them. Like tofu, they take on flavor brilliantly, and when cooked, they offer their own savory umami taste to any dish. Portobello mushrooms are well known for being hearty and "meaty"—I use them in a simple mushroom burger recipe (page 82)—but I also love trumpet and oyster mushrooms for their meaty texture. They can be sliced and added to any dish that normally contains beef or chicken.

I always have cremini mushrooms in my fridge because they are so versatile. Creminis can be sliced and added to anything from soups to casseroles, and when finely chopped, they can even be used in place of ground beef in a Bolognese sauce.

My little trick to bring out the meaty flavor of mushrooms is to add a splash of soy sauce when sautéing them. Give it a try—it works wonders!

Legumes

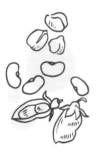

Other than green peas and the occasional lima bean, legumes are not something I grew up eating on a regular basis. These days, I have really come to appreciate beans of all shapes and sizes, from chickpeas to black beans to soybeans, and I always make sure to keep some stocked in my pantry.

Then there are lentils. Growing up, I associated lentils with soup and never thought much more about them. But since I began cooking more with lentils, I have grown to appreciate how they are a wonderful meat substitute. If you're looking for a swap for ground meat, cooked lentils are an easy way to go! They are already high in protein, plus they have a similar hearty texture. I use them to lessen the meat in my Lentil Pulled Pork Sandwiches (page 102), and I love how they lighten up the dish.

Cauliflower

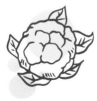

Cauliflower steaks may have been the world's introduction to cauliflower as a meat substitute, but aside from standing in for a filet, cauliflower has proven to be a versatile vegetable for other uses. Try my Buffalo Cauliflower "Wings" (page 74) for an indulgent snack, make Cauliflower Tacos (page 72) for taco Tuesday, or use cauliflower rice to stand in for ground meat in a filling. This cruciferous powerhouse is always satisfying.

Eggplant

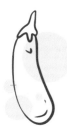

Eggplant is another food chameleon that makes an amazing meat substitute. Think of eggplant parmigiana. When it is breaded, fried, and smothered with marinara sauce and mozzarella cheese, I personally prefer eggplant parm to chicken parm any day of the week! Eggplant is sturdy enough for grilling and sautéing but also works beautifully in hearty sauces.

Like tofu, eggplant is a sponge to flavor, and you can use different varieties to get the results you want. Use hearty Italian globe eggplants for stuffing and roasting. Slender Chinese and Japanese eggplants are perfectly suited for sautéing and grilling.

Jackfruit

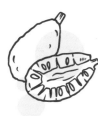

Jackfruit is native to Southeast Asia, and since I grew up in a Filipino-American household, my love for jackfruit is rooted in its use in sweet desserts and snacks. When I learned of jackfruit being used for savory dishes, I really had to reframe it in my mind! That said, I have grown to appreciate its use in vegetarian cooking. Because of its shredded meatlike texture and bland flavor, it can be used in so many ways. These days, jackfruit tacos make a regular appearance on my family table. Try it as pulled "pork," as a filling for dumplings, in a salad, and more!

Little Bites, Big Flavor

We miss two main things when we eat less meat: flavor and satisfaction (not feeling full). I combat this with the strategic use of small amounts of ingredients that deliver both. I call these "flavor bombs," and a little goes a long way to make a dish seem complete.

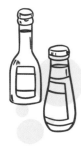

Umami

You may be familiar with the term *umami*, which is often described as the fifth taste, after sweet, sour, bitter, and salty. Umami is what gives food a meaty, savory flavor. Think of a flavorful bone broth, a delicious aged cheese, or a dish that includes a touch of fish sauce. It rounds out the palate, boosts flavor, and makes a meal more satisfying.

We can harness umami to make plant-forward dishes more flavorful, and it's all about stocking the pantry with flavor bombs! Soy sauce and fish sauce are extremely strong in umami, so I often use them in place of salt. Black bean sauce, miso paste, Worcestershire sauce, and anchovy paste are refrigerator staples that can instantly elevate a dish. It's amazing how a little dollop of one of these staples can add so much flavor.

A touch of pancetta, prosciutto, or bacon gives a dish the saltiness it needs without making it heavy. Sharp, pungent cheeses such as extra-sharp cheddar, Gruyère, feta, and Gorgonzola are much better for adding saltiness and fat than milder cheeses like Monterey Jack.

When cooked, mushrooms release a lovely umami flavor. If you're looking for more umami punch, opt for dark mushrooms such as cremini or morel mushrooms or, even better, dried ones. I keep dried shiitake mushrooms in my pantry so I can easily add flavor to gravies, broths, and more. Using mushrooms is a wonderful way to get that deep umami flavor without the fat or cholesterol in meat or cheese.

Spice

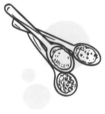

Adding heat to a dish is a simple yet effective way to add a kick, leaving you much more satisfied. If you love spice, then you know what I mean! Essentials to keep on hand include chili oil, chipotles in adobo sauce, garam masala, gochujang, harissa, Sriracha sauce, and Thai red curry paste. If you are averse to spice, try adding small amounts to your cooking—you might find you can tolerate it and grow to crave it.

Acidity

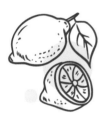

When a dish tastes flat, chances are it needs a touch of acidity. It's amazing what a squeeze of lemon or lime juice can do to brighten a meal! I also keep a collection of vinegars in my pantry—adding just a splash of vinegar to a soup, for example, rounds out the broth and really livens it up.

Fresh Herbs and Alliums

Fresh, fragrant herbs make a world of difference in cooking—you will see that I am huge fan of basil, cilantro, dill, and parsley, along with pungent alliums like garlic and green onions. They add flavor and elevate a dish instantly.

Stocking the Pantry for Freshness

When it comes to eating plant-forward, you might assume that fresh produce is best. The truth is, you can stock the pantry for freshness, ensuring that a healthy, nourishing meal is always at your fingertips.

If you've shied away from canned vegetables, I am here to encourage you to rethink this position. I used to assume that canned vegetables were not as fresh as the real thing, but the truth is, canned vegetables are picked at their peak, preserving nutrients and flavor.

One prime example is canned tomatoes. Fresh tomatoes must be picked a few days before they are fully ripe to account for shipping and transport time, whereas canned tomatoes can be picked at the point of peak ripeness for canning, so I often reach for canned tomatoes, depending on the recipe.

That said, certain vegetables seem to work better than others for canning. Besides tomatoes, I love to stock up on canned corn, peas, olives, and green beans. While technically not a vegetable, canned beans are also a pantry staple. The only caveat is to read the labels—watch out for added sodium or sugar, and if there is any added salt, rinse and drain the vegetables or beans before using.

When you hear the word *pantry,* you might think of canned goods and dry goods such as pasta, but I also like to think of the fridge and freezer. I lump this in as part of my "pantry" since it's all about stocking the kitchen with essentials.

Let's start with the freezer. Again, frozen vegetables are wonderful to keep on hand, and in some ways, they offer more flexibility than canned vegetables. Besides keeping the quintessential mixed vegetables on hand, I love having frozen peas, corn, edamame, kale, broccoli, zucchini noodles, pasta, and grains. I also like to peel fresh ginger, slice it, and freeze it—ready to pop into any dish!

As for the refrigerator, I like to make sure it's stocked with vegetables that are hardy and long-lasting, depending on the season. Broccoli and cauliflower, cabbage and Brussels sprouts, winter squash, carrots and celery, and kale do quite well (hurray for winter vegetables!). Citrus, green onions, and fresh herbs are a must. I always keep certain ingredients on hand for flavor, such as pancetta, prosciutto, cheeses like feta and sharp cheddar, and of course, unsalted butter.

Helpful Tools

I try my best to create recipes that don't require many special tools. However, in addition to basics like mixing bowls, measuring tools, a good knife or two, and some pots and pans, there are a few tools that I highly recommend and consider essential to any kitchen.

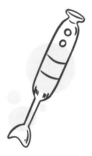

Blender/Immersion Blender

A blender is a workhorse in my kitchen. I use mine daily—from morning smoothies to blending sauces and dressings, I truly couldn't live without it. I also have an immersion blender (pictured), which is especially handy for puréeing soups and finessing the texture of a dish. It's not necessary to have both types, but I recommend having some kind of blender!

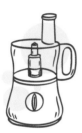

Food Processor

Food processors are very similar to blenders, but rather than liquids, food processors are perfect for more solid foods. You can shred, slice, and finely chop food with a food processor, saving time and effort. It can even mix dough. Most of the things a food processor does, you can do by hand with a knife, of course, but it really makes life in the kitchen easier!

Spiralizer

You won't use a spiralizer every day, but it comes in handy for making noodles from vegetables, and if that encourages you to eat more veggies, then I think it's a win! These days, you can find prespiralized vegetables at the grocery store, but why pay more when you can do it yourself at home?

Transforming Leftovers

Ah, leftovers. Some people loathe them, while others love them. Me? I'm a huge fan. Having leftovers means not only that I have a ready-made meal for lunch the next day, but also that I have the opportunity to invent a whole new meal, saving time and money as well. I embrace leftovers and use them to my advantage.

Let's start with the most common leftover: roast chicken. The possibilities are endless. You can make a delicious broth from the carcass and use the leftover meat in so many applications. In this book, you'll find several recipes in which you can use leftover chicken, such as the Curry Chicken Salad Bowls (page 158) and the Chicken, Mushroom, and Corn Tetrazzini (page 208).

Leftover roasted vegetables can be used in so many ways, too! Make a large batch of the roasted veggies for Roasted Vegetable Breakfast Burritos (page 42), and you can use the extras for a Roasted Vegetable Galette (page 86)—or vice versa. You could even throw them into a vegetable ragout. The same goes for the roasted squash used in the Roasted Winter Squash, Kale, and Turkey Bacon Pizza (page 94) and the Winter Squash Quinoa Salad (page 144).

My fridge often holds some kind of leftover rice or grain, which is one of the easiest types of food to transform. Leftover quinoa is perfect for a salad or stuffed into mushrooms or peppers. Extra barley makes it easier to throw together dishes like my Vegetable Beef and Barley Soup (page 122) or Skirt Steak with Peppers, Onions, and Barley (page 212).

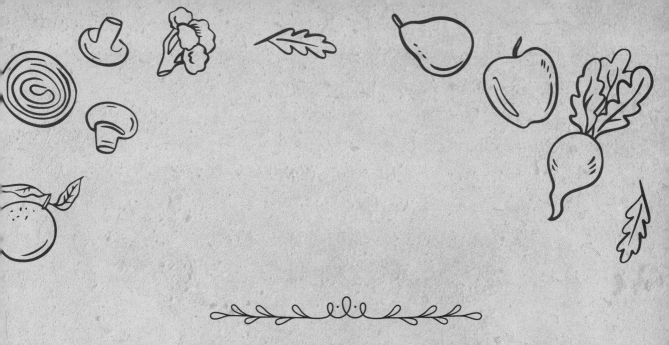

RECIPES

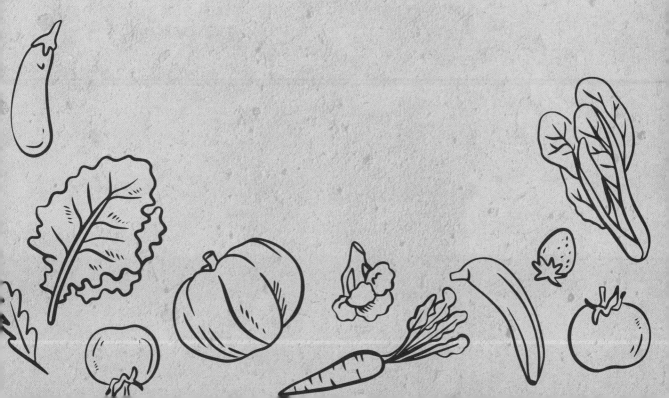

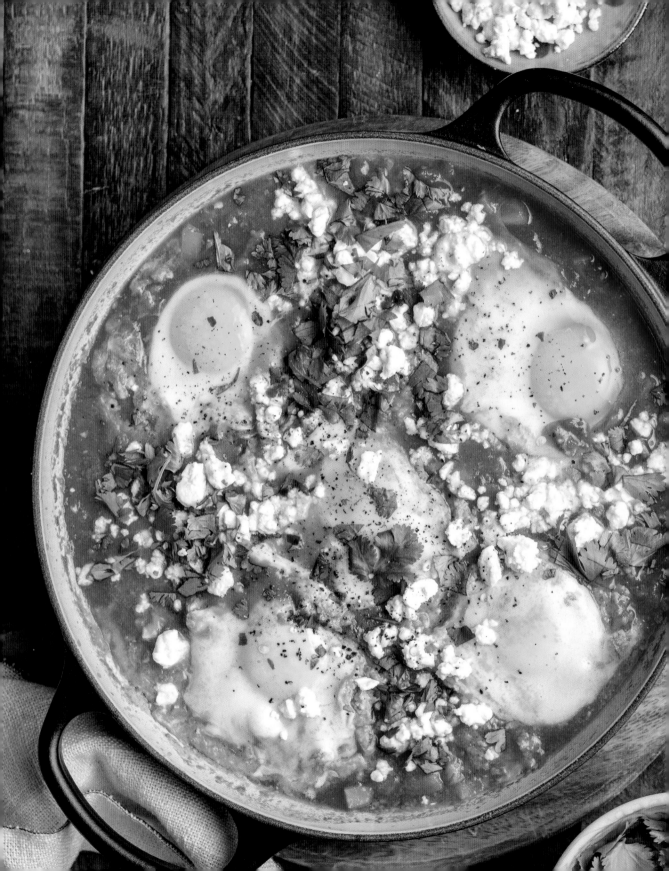

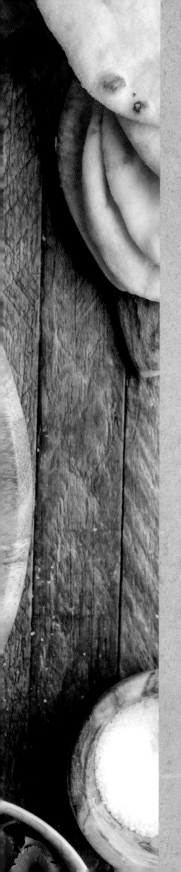

Breakfasts

Savory Veggie Waffles *with* Mushroom Gravy

Yield: 4 servings

Prep Time: 15 minutes

Cook Time: 25 minutes

Are you a sweet or a savory person? I am willing to bet that even if you are on team sweet, this zucchini cheddar version will convince you that savory waffles for breakfast are a good idea! I love dipping them in mushroom gravy, but they're also incredible with a side of eggs and bacon.

FOR THE GRAVY:

2 tablespoons unsalted butter

8 ounces cremini mushrooms, sliced

1 clove garlic, minced

1 teaspoon soy sauce

2 tablespoons all-purpose flour

1¼ cups vegetable stock

Kosher salt and freshly ground black pepper

FOR THE WAFFLES:

2 cups coarsely shredded zucchini (about 2 medium zucchini), squeezed dry

¼ cup coarsely shredded yellow onions, squeezed dry

2 large eggs, lightly beaten

⅔ cup shredded cheddar cheese

¼ cup chopped green onions

¼ cup all-purpose flour

1 teaspoon baking powder

1 teaspoon kosher salt

½ teaspoon freshly ground black pepper

Extra-virgin olive oil, for the waffle iron

Make the gravy:

1. Melt the butter in a medium saucepan over medium heat. Add the mushrooms and garlic and cook for 5 to 10 minutes, until the mushrooms are tender. Season with the soy sauce.

2. Stir in the flour and cook for another 1 to 2 minutes, just to toast the flour.

3. Mix in the vegetable stock and bring to a boil, whisking periodically. Lower the heat to a simmer and cook until the gravy has thickened to your desired consistency.

4. Season to taste with salt and pepper. Keep warm until ready to serve.

Make the waffles:

5. Preheat a waffle iron to the high setting. If you will not be serving the waffles immediately, preheat the oven to 175°F, place an ovenproof wire cooling rack in a sheet pan, and set the pan in the center of the oven.

6. Mix the zucchini, onions, and eggs in a large bowl until combined. Stir in the cheese and green onions.

7. In a small bowl, whisk together the flour, baking powder, salt, and pepper. Add to the zucchini mixture, mixing until just combined. If the batter is too runny, mix in more flour.

8. Lightly brush some olive oil onto the plates of the waffle iron, then pour a scant ½ cup of batter into each cavity (depending on the size of your waffle iron). Cook for 5 to 7 minutes, or until the waffles are golden and crispy on the outside. If not serving right away, transfer the waffles to the cooling rack in the oven (do not stack them, as this would make them soggy). Serve with the gravy.

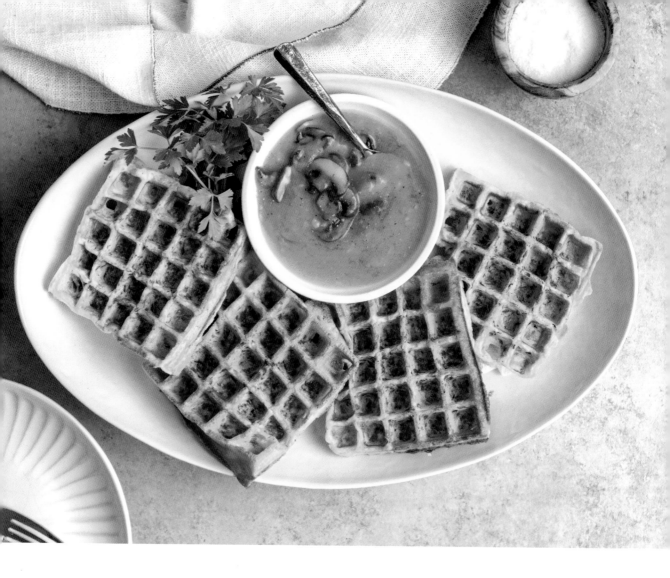

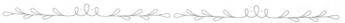

NOTES

This recipe makes 4 waffles. I find that 1 waffle per person is quite filling, especially when served with gravy or a side of eggs.

Cooked and fully cooled waffles can be stored in the refrigerator for up to 3 days or frozen for longer. To freeze, place a layer of parchment or wax paper between the waffles and store in a freezer bag or resealable container in the freezer for up to 3 months.

To reheat the waffles, preheat the oven to 350°F. Lay the waffles in a single layer on a sheet pan and bake for 10 to 15 minutes, or until heated through.

Kale *and* Ham Frittata

Yield: 4 servings
Prep Time: 10 minutes
Cook Time: 20 minutes

I can't help but think of my mom whenever I make this recipe! Whenever she was pressed for time or inspiration, and no matter what ingredients she had in the refrigerator, she could always whip up a frittata. Not only was it a great way to use up extra produce, but it was also the perfect way to get us kids to eat more veggies! This kale and ham frittata is a hearty way to start the day, but it's also delicious for lunch or dinner, especially when served with a side salad. My Chickpea Summer Salad on page 136 is a great choice.

2 tablespoons extra-virgin olive oil

⅓ cup finely chopped yellow onions

1½ cups chopped kale

4 ounces thinly sliced deli ham, cut into 2-inch ribbons

6 large eggs

2 tablespoons unsweetened, unflavored milk (coconut, almond, or dairy)

½ teaspoon kosher salt

Pinch of freshly ground black pepper

½ cup crumbled feta cheese

1. Preheat the oven to 400°F with a rack placed in the center of the oven.

2. Heat the olive oil in an 8-inch cast-iron or other ovenproof nonstick skillet over medium heat. Swirl the pan to coat the bottom and sides with the oil. Add the onions and cook until wilted and translucent, about 3 minutes. Stir in the kale and ham and cook for 2 minutes to wilt the kale.

3. Quickly whisk together the eggs, milk, salt, and pepper, then pour the mixture into the skillet. Using a rubber spatula, push the edges of the eggs toward the center of the pan, stirring around the curds as they form.

4. Gently stir in the cheese while the eggs are still very loose with some curds.

5. Transfer the skillet to the oven and bake for 10 to 15 minutes, or until the frittata is lofty, the eggs are set, and a knife comes out clean when inserted in the center.

6. Remove from the oven and let stand for 3 minutes before slicing and serving.

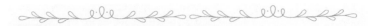

NOTE

Frittatas are a great make-ahead meal. They keep well in the refrigerator, making them perfect for busy mornings. I like to slice up the frittata after it cools and then refrigerate the slices in an airtight container for a grab-and-go breakfast. It can be reheated in the microwave or eaten at room temperature.

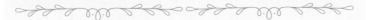

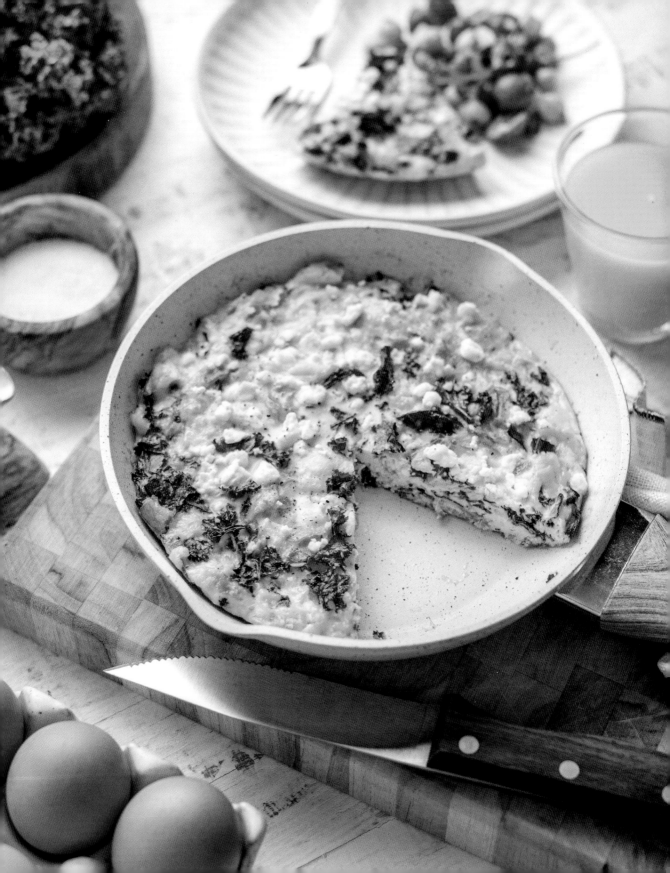

Savory Zucchini Cheddar Muffins

Yield: 12 muffins

Prep Time: 10 minutes

Cook Time: 21 minutes

Muffins are a delicious way to brighten up any morning, and these savory muffins are my favorite way to sneak in extra veggies for breakfast. (Who can resist anything with cheese?) Not only will extra muffins keep for those busy mornings, but they're also perfect for afternoon snacking or serving with a hearty soup at dinnertime.

3 cups all-purpose flour

3 tablespoons granulated sugar

1 tablespoon plus 1 teaspoon baking powder

½ teaspoon baking soda

1 teaspoon kosher salt

1 teaspoon garlic powder

1 teaspoon onion powder

½ teaspoon freshly ground black pepper

1½ cups shredded extra-sharp cheddar cheese

½ cup grated Parmigiano-Reggiano cheese

⅓ cup sliced green onions

4 cups shredded zucchini (about 4 medium zucchini) (see Notes)

4 large eggs, lightly beaten

⅔ cup extra-virgin olive oil

¼ cup buttermilk

1. Preheat the oven to 425°F with a rack placed in the upper third of the oven. Line a 12-cup muffin pan with cupcake liners or lightly grease it with baking spray. Set aside.

2. In a large bowl, whisk together the flour, sugar, baking powder, baking soda, salt, garlic powder, onion powder, and pepper. Stir in the cheeses and green onions.

3. In a separate bowl, mix the zucchini, eggs, olive oil, and buttermilk until well blended. Add the zucchini mixture to the dry ingredients and stir until just combined. Do not overmix.

4. Divide the batter evenly among the prepared muffin cups, filling each nearly to the top. Bake for 6 minutes, then lower the oven temperature to 350°F and bake for another 15 minutes, or until a toothpick inserted into the center of a muffin comes out clean and the tops are golden and firm to the touch.

5. Remove from the oven, allow the muffins to cool in the pan for 5 minutes, and then transfer them to a wire rack to cool for at least 10 more minutes before serving. Enjoy warm or at room temperature.

6. Store cooled muffins between two layers of paper towels in an airtight container in the refrigerator, where they will keep for 3 to 4 days. They can also be frozen in an airtight freezer-safe container for up to 3 months. Defrost the muffins in the refrigerator overnight before reheating (see Notes).

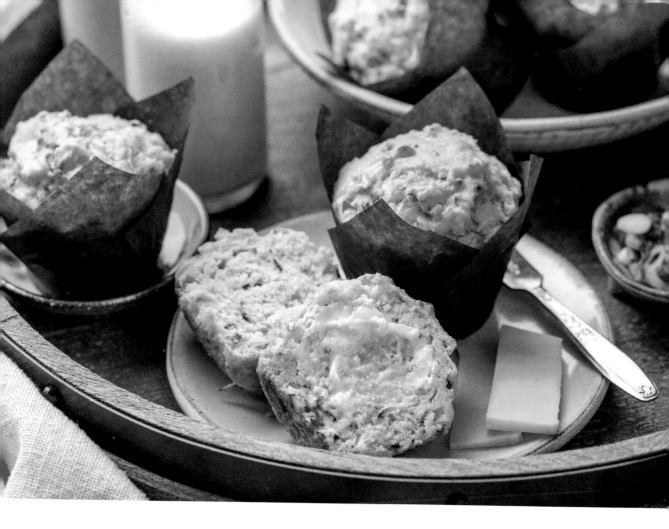

NOTES

The quality of the cheese really makes a difference in these muffins! Be sure to use a good-quality Parmesan and an extra-sharp cheddar so that you can really taste the flavor (if you can find an aged cheddar, even better). I highly recommend Parmigiano-Reggiano cheese and Tillamook Extra Sharp Cheddar (Vintage if you can find it).

If you notice that the shredded zucchini is especially liquid-y, take the time to lightly press it between some clean paper towels to remove any excess moisture. Admittedly, I usually skip this step when pinched for time, but if the zucchini is wetter than usual, I do recommend that you take the time to do so.

The muffins can be reheated in a preheated 350°F oven for about 10 minutes or in the microwave for 20 seconds.

Shakshuka *with* Breakfast Sausage

Yield: 5 servings
Prep Time: 10 minutes
Cook Time: 30 minutes

Shakshuka may also be known as "eggs in hell," but there's something heavenly about eggs poached in a fiery tomato sauce. This classic gets an extra breakfast-y boost with breakfast sausage, and it's often a favorite in my family when we're craving breakfast for dinner. Don't forget the pita bread, which is perfect for sopping up the delicious sauce!

1 tablespoon extra-virgin olive oil

½ cup finely chopped yellow onions

2½ teaspoons minced garlic (about 3 cloves)

Kosher salt and freshly ground black pepper

7 ounces bulk pork breakfast sausage (not in casings)

1 cup diced red or orange bell peppers

1 (28-ounce) can whole San Marzano tomatoes

1½ tablespoons harissa

2 teaspoons tomato paste

2 teaspoons smoked paprika

1 teaspoon ground cumin

5 large eggs

Red pepper flakes

½ cup roughly chopped fresh cilantro

¼ cup crumbled feta cheese

Pita bread, for serving

1. Heat the olive oil in a 3-quart sauté pan over medium-low heat. Add the onions and garlic and season lightly with a pinch each of salt and pepper. Cook until the onions are translucent, about 3 minutes.

2. Increase the heat to medium-high. Add the sausage and bell peppers, breaking up the sausage into bits with a wooden spoon, and cook for another 5 to 7 minutes, or until the sausage is nearly cooked and the bell peppers are beginning to soften.

3. Meanwhile, using an immersion blender or a wooden spoon, crush the tomatoes in their juice until they are broken down but still chunky.

4. To the sausage mixture, add the crushed tomatoes, harissa, tomato paste, smoked paprika, cumin, and ½ teaspoon of salt. Stir to combine and cook for another 5 minutes to allow the flavors to develop.

5. Use the back of a spoon to create little pockets in the sauce, then gently break an egg into each pocket. Season the eggs with salt, pepper, and red pepper flakes, spooning a little sauce onto the whites around the edges of the eggs.

6. Cover and reduce the heat to low; let simmer until the egg whites are set and the yolks are cooked to your desired doneness, 12 to 15 minutes.

7. Top with the cilantro and feta cheese. Serve immediately with pita bread on the side.

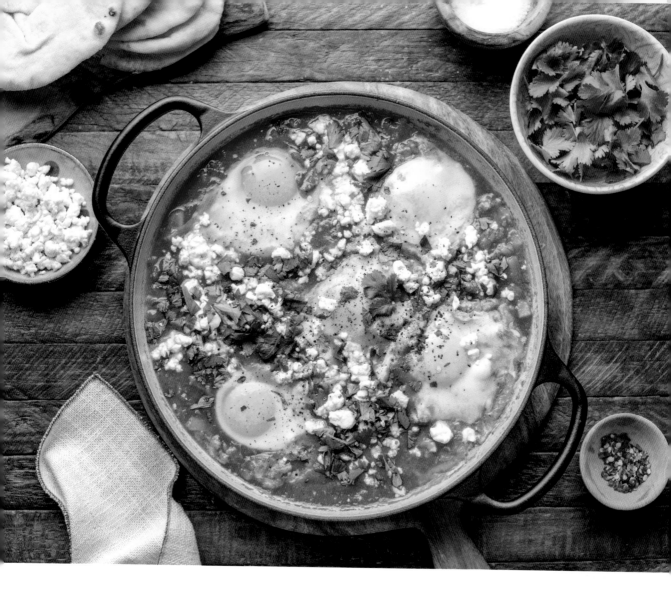

NOTES

Cooking shakshuka in a cast-iron skillet is in vogue, but unless your skillet is truly well seasoned, I don't recommend it. Due to the acidity of the tomato sauce, cooking shakshuka in a cast-iron skillet that hasn't been seasoned adequately can strip the seasoning and give the dish a metallic taste. Instead, opt for enameled cast iron or stainless-steel cookware.

Shakshuka is traditionally made without meat. If you prefer a meatless version, simply omit the breakfast sausage—it will be just as delicious!

Yield: 8 to 10 servings

Prep Time: 10 minutes, plus 1 hour to rest

Cook Time: 50 minutes

Breakfast Strata

Breakfast casseroles are a godsend when you've got to feed a crowd in the morning. This strata is essentially a savory bread pudding, combining all the best parts of breakfast into one dish!

6 large eggs

1½ cups whole milk

¾ teaspoon kosher salt

½ teaspoon paprika

¼ teaspoon freshly ground black pepper

1½ cups tender greens, such as spinach or baby kale

1 cup diced mushrooms (any type)

1 cup cherry tomatoes, halved

¼ cup finely diced red onions

½ cup chopped ham

6 ounces rustic French bread, cut into 1-inch pieces (about 3 cups)

¾ cup shredded cheddar cheese

¾ cup shredded Havarti cheese

¼ cup grated Parmigiano-Reggiano cheese, plus more for garnish

1 tablespoon chopped flat-leaf parsley, for garnish (optional)

1. Grease a 1½-quart baking dish with butter. Set aside.

2. In a large bowl, whisk the eggs, milk, salt, paprika, and pepper until combined. Fold in the greens, mushrooms, tomatoes, red onions, ham, bread, and cheddar and Havarti cheeses. Pour the mixture into the baking dish and top with the Parmigiano-Reggiano cheese. Cover the baking dish with plastic wrap and set in the refrigerator to rest for 1 hour or overnight.

3. When ready to bake, preheat the oven to 350°F with a rack placed in the center of the oven. Remove the strata from the refrigerator to rest at room temperature while the oven preheats.

4. Remove the plastic wrap, cover the strata with foil, and bake for 35 minutes. Uncover and bake for another 15 minutes, or until it is puffed and set in the center. Let rest for 5 minutes before slicing. Garnish with Parmigiano-Reggiano and the parsley, if desired. Enjoy warm.

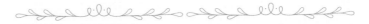

NOTE

Like any bread pudding, strata is even better when the bread has had time to soak in the custard, making it ideal to prep the night before baking.

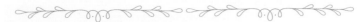

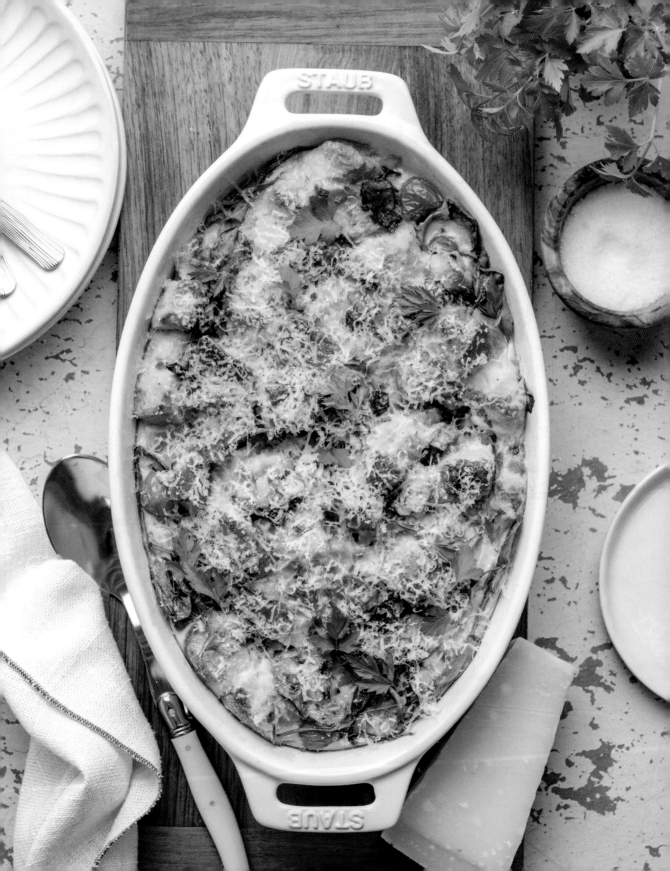

Berry Baked Oatmeal

Yield: 12 servings

Prep Time: 10 minutes

Cook Time: 45 minutes

Every day starts with oatmeal at my house. Hearty and cozy, it keeps us fueled for busy mornings. Once in a while, I love to trade my bowl for a slice of baked oatmeal—it's easy to make in advance and keeps for days in the refrigerator, making mornings even easier. Bonus: you can even have it for dessert! Dollop some whipped cream or ice cream on top and make it a treat.

2 cups rolled oats

⅓ cup brown sugar

1½ teaspoons ground cinnamon

1 teaspoon baking powder

½ teaspoon kosher salt

3 cups mixed berries, chopped if large, divided

1 cup chopped raw pecans, divided

1 cup unsweetened, unflavored milk (coconut, almond, or dairy)

2 large eggs

¼ cup melted (but not hot) coconut oil or unsalted butter, plus more for the pan

2 teaspoons vanilla extract

TOPPINGS (OPTIONAL):

Chia seeds

Shelled hemp seeds (aka hemp hearts)

Nuts

Maple syrup

1. Preheat the oven to 350°F with a rack placed in the upper third of the oven. Lightly grease a 9-inch pie pan with coconut oil or butter.

2. In a large bowl, mix together the oats, brown sugar, cinnamon, baking powder, and salt. Gently toss in 2½ cups of the berries and ½ cup of the pecans.

3. In a small bowl, whisk together the milk, eggs, coconut oil, and vanilla until blended. Gently stir the milk mixture into the oat mixture, taking care not to crush the berries.

4. Transfer the mixture to the prepared pie pan. Bake for 45 minutes, or until the oats are set, the top is browned, and the berries are bubbling.

5. Let the baked oatmeal cool and set for about 20 minutes.

6. Top the baked oatmeal with the remaining ½ cup of berries and ½ cup of pecans. Slice and serve with additional toppings, if desired. The oatmeal will keep, refrigerated, for up to 5 days. For longer storage, freeze slices in a freezer-safe container for up to 3 months.

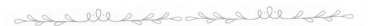

NOTE

Slices of baked oatmeal can be reheated in the microwave for about 45 seconds. I confess to eating leftovers cold, too, especially if I'm in a rush!

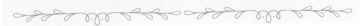

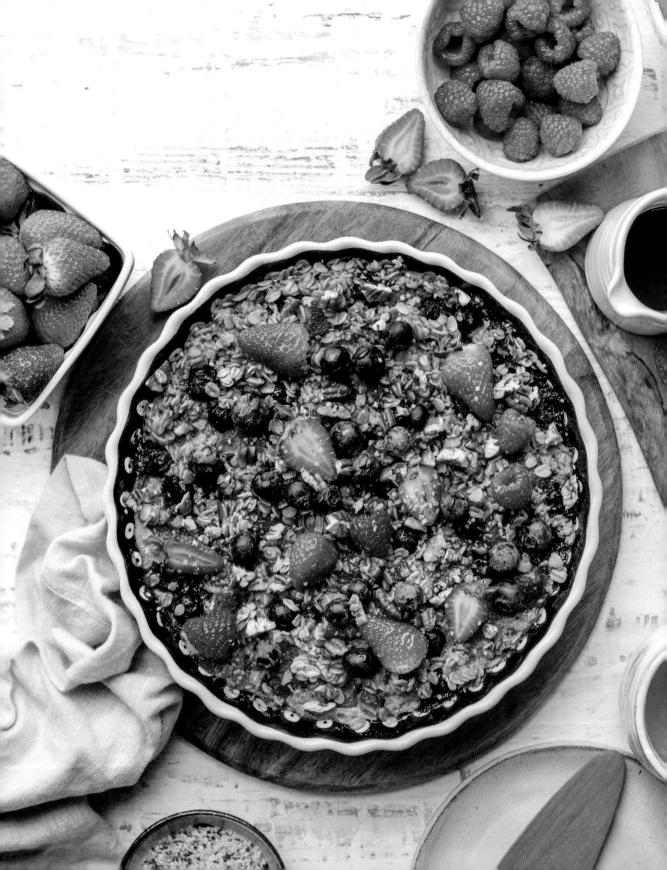

Breakfast Bibimbap

Yield: 4 servings
Prep Time: 15 minutes
Cook Time: 25 minutes

The first time I had bibimbap was at one of my favorite Korean restaurants in New York. I was just a little girl, but even then, I instantly thought it would be the perfect meal to start the day! Topped with an egg, this meat and vegetable–laden rice bowl reminds me of the egg-and-rice breakfasts my mom would make for us. So I say, why not enjoy it in the morning? This version uses ground beef instead of steak, which eliminates the need for marinating, and all the components can be made in advance. A rice bowl full of savory meat, lots of veggies, and an egg all mixed up with a spicy sauce is the ultimate way to start the day!

FOR THE BIBIMBAP SAUCE:

¼ cup gochujang paste

2 tablespoons mirin (sweet rice wine)

2 tablespoons unseasoned rice vinegar

2 tablespoons untoasted sesame oil (unrefined)

1 tablespoon soy sauce

2 teaspoons granulated sugar

2 cloves garlic, minced

FOR THE BEEF:

2 teaspoons extra-virgin olive oil

1 pound 85% lean ground beef

¼ cup peeled, grated Asian pear (aka apple pear)

2 green onions, thinly sliced

2 cloves garlic, minced

2 tablespoons gochujang paste

2 tablespoons soy sauce

1 tablespoon unseasoned rice vinegar

FOR THE BOWLS:

1 tablespoon plus 2 teaspoons extra-virgin olive oil, divided

½ cup shredded carrots

4 cups baby spinach

1 cup sliced shiitake mushrooms

Soy sauce or kosher salt

Freshly ground black pepper

4 large eggs

4 cups cooked white rice

¼ cup sliced green onions (white and green parts) (see Notes)

¼ cup kimchi

OPTIONAL GARNISHES:

1 cup shredded red cabbage

½ cucumber, sliced in half lengthwise, then into half-moons

¼ cup chopped fresh cilantro

1 tablespoon black and/or white sesame seeds

(recipe continues on page 37)

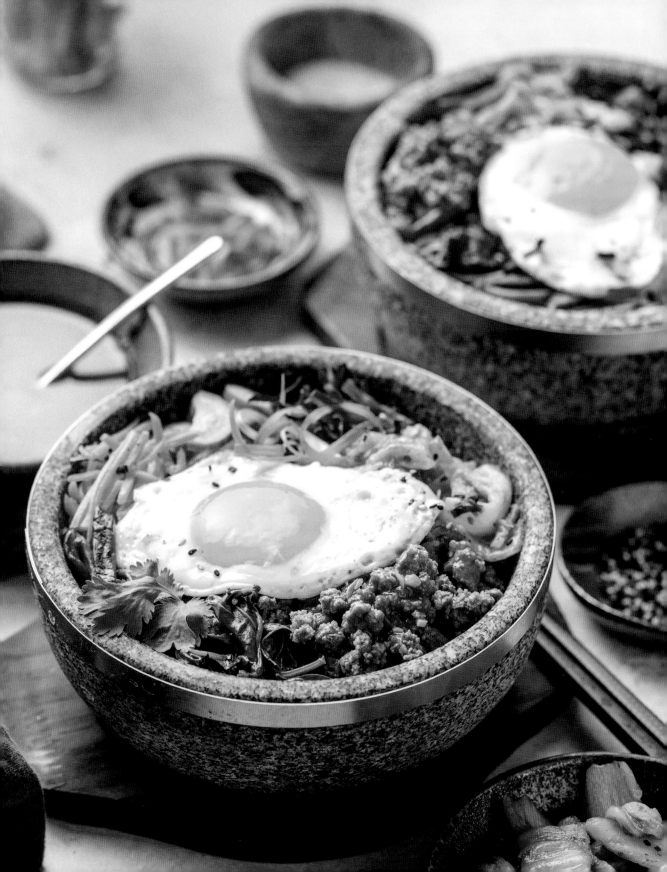

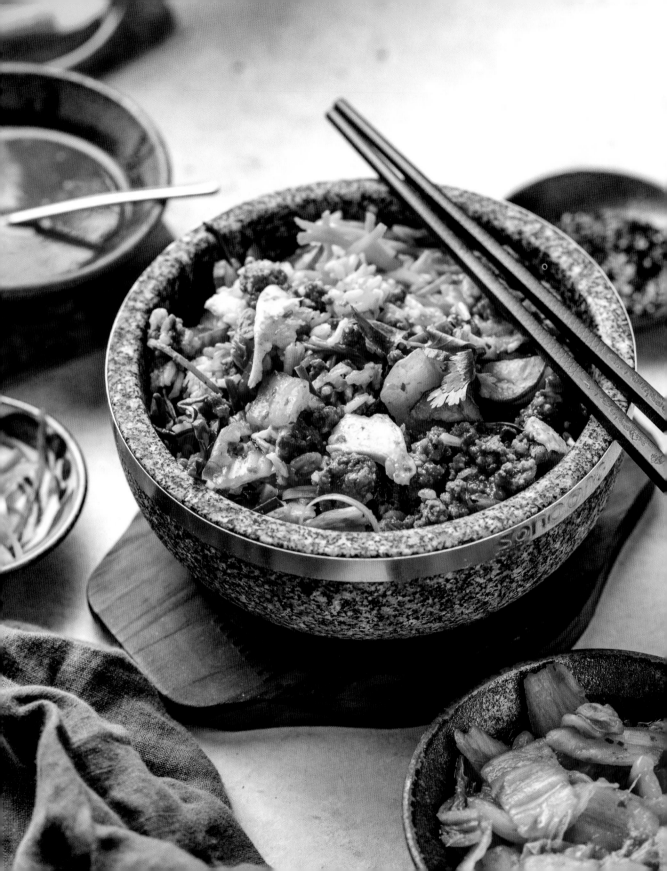

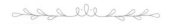

These days, it's easier to find Asian pears at the grocery store than it used to be. However, if you can't find any, you can substitute an Anjou or Bosc pear.

Gochujang is a Korean chili paste that can be found in the Asian section of the grocery store. It's a versatile ingredient, much like harissa or Sriracha sauce.

Looking to make the garnish a little prettier? Make green onion curls by slicing the green onion into 3-inch-long julienne strips. Immerse the strips in a bowl of ice water for about 10 minutes, until curled.

The components of this dish can be made in advance, making breakfast the next morning even simpler! Make the rice, sauce, beef, and vegetable toppings up to 2 days in advance, then reheat and build your bowls in the morning.

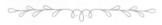

Make the sauce:

1. In a small bowl, whisk together the ingredients for the sauce. Set aside.

Make the beef:

2. Heat the olive oil in a 3-quart sauté pan over medium heat. Add the ground beef and use a wooden spoon to break it up into bits. Stir in the grated pear, green onions, garlic, gochujang paste, soy sauce, and vinegar. Cook for about 7 minutes, until the meat is fully cooked, then transfer to a bowl and set aside.

Make the bowls:

3. In the same pan you used for the beef, heat 1 tablespoon of the olive oil over medium heat. Working in batches, sauté the carrots, spinach, and mushrooms until the carrots are tender, the spinach is wilted, and the mushrooms are browned. Season with a few drops of soy sauce (or a pinch of salt) and a pinch of pepper.

4. Heat the remaining 2 teaspoons of olive oil in a medium nonstick skillet over low heat. Crack the eggs into the skillet, cover with a lid, and fry sunny-side-up for 2 minutes for runny yolks, or longer until the yolks are cooked to your liking. Season with salt and pepper to taste.

5. Place a cup of rice in each bowl. Divide the beef and vegetables among the bowls and top each with an egg, one-quarter each of the green onions and kimchi, and a drizzle of the sauce. If desired, garnish with red cabbage, cucumber, cilantro, and/or sesame seeds. Serve with additional sauce. To eat, stir the ingredients well and enjoy!

Cauliflower Steak and *Eggs*

Yield: 4 servings

Prep Time: 10 minutes

Cook Time: 20 minutes

There's nothing heartier than steak and eggs for breakfast, but when you need to lighten things up, why not try cauliflower steaks? To brighten things further, I serve the "steak" and eggs with a zingy herb sauce inspired by one of my favorite combinations: steak and chimichurri.

FOR THE HERB SAUCE:

⅓ cup extra-virgin olive oil

½ cup chopped fresh cilantro

¼ cup minced red onions

3 tablespoons sherry vinegar

2 teaspoons minced garlic (2 to 3 cloves)

1 teaspoon red pepper flakes

½ teaspoon kosher salt

⅛ teaspoon cayenne pepper

⅛ teaspoon freshly ground black pepper

FOR THE CAULIFLOWER STEAK AND EGGS:

2 small heads cauliflower

3 tablespoons plus 2 teaspoons extra-virgin olive oil, divided

Steak seasoning

Kosher salt and freshly ground black pepper

4 large eggs

1. Preheat the oven to 350°F with a rack placed in the center of the oven.

Make the sauce:

2. In a small bowl, stir together the ingredients for the sauce. Set aside.

Make the cauliflower steaks:

3. Remove and discard the tough leaves from the base of one of the cauliflower heads; you can leave the tender leaves in place. Trim the stem to create a stable base for the cauliflower. Turn the cauliflower onto the flat base, floret side up. Slice the head of cauliflower in half, straight through the stem; then, working from the center cut, slice a 1¼-inch-thick steak from each half. Reserve the extra florets for another recipe. Repeat with the other cauliflower head to make 4 steaks.

4. Brush the steaks on both sides with 2 tablespoons of the olive oil and season liberally with steak seasoning, salt, and pepper.

5. Heat an extra-large ovenproof skillet over medium-high heat. Pour 1 tablespoon of the olive oil into the pan and let it heat up, then add the cauliflower steaks. Fry for about 4 minutes, until the steaks are turning golden brown. Flip the cauliflower, transfer the skillet to the oven, and roast for 12 to 15 minutes, until the stems are tender when you insert a sharp paring knife. *Note:* I use a 15¾-inch skillet to fry the steaks all at once without crowding them. If your skillet isn't large enough for all of the cauliflower steaks, fry them in batches and transfer them to a sheet pan before roasting in the oven.

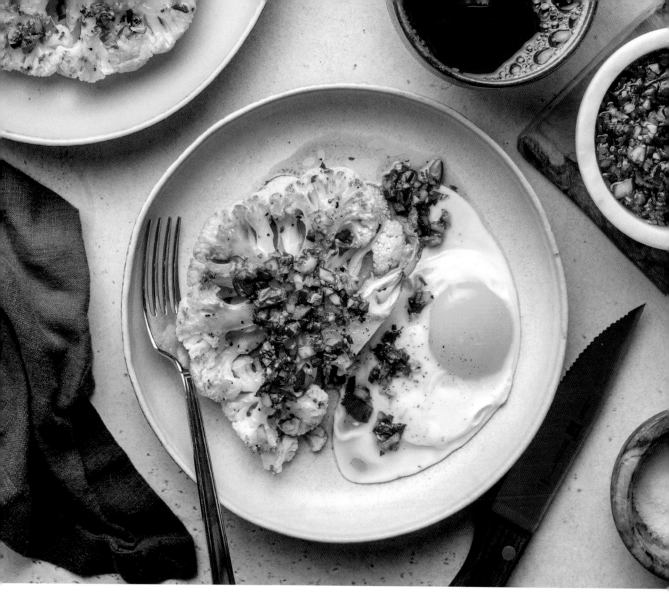

NOTE

The herb sauce can be made up to 48 hours in advance but is best if used within 24 hours.

Make the eggs:

6. When the cauliflower is nearly done, prepare the eggs: Heat the remaining 2 teaspoons of olive oil in a medium nonstick skillet over low heat. Crack the eggs into the pan, cover with a lid, and fry for 2 minutes for sunny-side-up eggs with runny yolks, or longer until the yolks are cooked to your liking. Season with salt and pepper to taste.

Assembly:

7. To serve, place a cauliflower steak on each plate, add an egg, and drizzle with herb sauce.

Chipotle Huevos Rancheros

Yield: 4 servings

Prep Time: 10 minutes

Cook Time: 30 minutes

I have certain go-to dishes when I go out for breakfast and brunch, and huevos rancheros is one of them. But when making it at home is so simple, why bother going out? This version, chock-full of hearty beans, gets a flavor boost from turkey bacon and spicy chipotle powder. The bean topping is delicious for more than breakfast—we love using it in burritos, spooned onto sweet potatoes, or as a simple side dish. But of course, serve it with an egg over tortillas, and you have an incredible breakfast!

1 tablespoon plus 2 teaspoons extra-virgin olive oil, divided

½ cup finely chopped yellow onions

2 slices turkey bacon, chopped into ¼-inch pieces

1 (15-ounce) can black beans, drained and rinsed

½ cup corn kernels (see Notes)

½ cup chopped orange or red bell peppers

1 teaspoon minced garlic

½ teaspoon chipotle powder (see Notes)

¼ teaspoon ground cumin

¼ teaspoon paprika

½ cup chicken stock

½ teaspoon Worcestershire sauce

Kosher salt and freshly ground black pepper

4 (4½-inch) corn tortillas

4 large eggs

FOR GARNISH:

½ cup crumbled Cotija or feta cheese

½ cup chopped fresh cilantro

1 avocado, pitted, peeled, and sliced

¼ cup salsa, plus more for serving if desired

1. Heat 1 tablespoon of the olive oil in a medium skillet over medium-low heat. Add the onions and cook until translucent, about 4 minutes.

2. Stir in the bacon, black beans, corn, bell peppers, garlic, chipotle powder, cumin, paprika, chicken stock, and Worcestershire sauce. Reduce the heat to low and simmer for 7 to 10 minutes, or until the mixture has thickened. Season with salt and pepper to taste.

3. While the beans are cooking, heat a medium nonstick skillet over medium heat. One by one, warm the tortillas for 1 to 2 minutes on each side. Cover to keep warm and set aside.

4. Heat the remaining 2 teaspoons of olive oil in the nonstick skillet over low heat. Crack the eggs into the skillet, cover with a lid, and fry sunny-side-up for 2 minutes for runny yolks, or longer until the yolks are cooked to your liking. Season with salt and pepper to taste.

5. To serve, place a tortilla on each plate. Top with the bean and corn mixture and an egg. Garnish with the cheese, cilantro, avocado slices, and/or salsa, if desired.

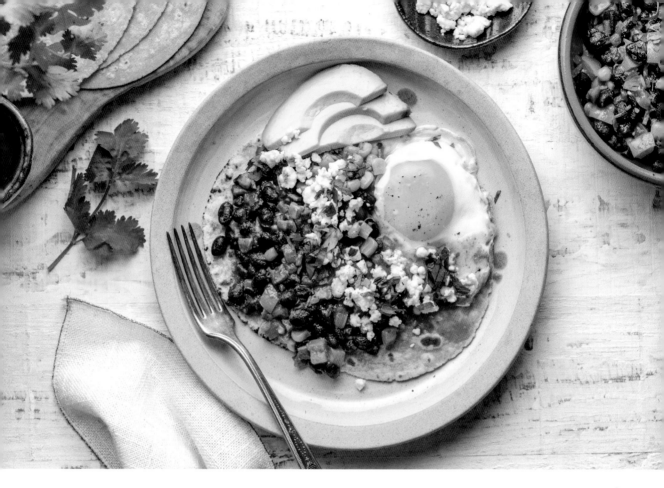

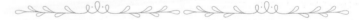

NOTES

A tortilla warmer is handy, but another way to keep tortillas nice and toasty is to place them on a sheet pan in a 125°F oven while you prepare the rest of the dish.

Feeling extra hungry? Consider serving 2 tortillas per serving for a heartier breakfast.

Corn adds a little sweetness to the dish—frozen kernels are easy to keep on hand and are perfect for dishes like this one. Feel free to use fresh, canned, or frozen corn kernels; regardless of the type, the cooking time is the same. If you use frozen corn kernels, you can add them straight into the pan from the freezer! If using fresh, you'll need 1 ear of corn for this quantity of kernels.

This amount of chipotle powder gives the dish a medium level of spiciness. If you are sensitive to spiciness, use less, to taste—and of course, if you prefer more kick, use more chipotle powder!

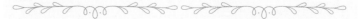

Roasted Vegetable Breakfast Burritos

Yield: 4 servings

Prep Time: 20 minutes

Cook Time: 25 minutes

Breakfast burritos are a thing at our house. They're a go-to for breakfast, of course, but also for lunch and even dinner, because who doesn't love an eggy burrito, as my kids call it? I especially love making them with roasted vegetables for a well-balanced start to the day.

FOR THE ROASTED VEGETABLES:

1½ cups diced butternut squash

1 cup broccoli florets

1 cup quartered cremini or white mushrooms

1 cup diced yellow squash

1 cup diced zucchini

½ cup diced red onions

½ cup roughly chopped red bell peppers

2 cloves garlic, minced

2 tablespoons extra-virgin olive oil

1 teaspoon herbes de Provence

Kosher salt and freshly ground black pepper

FOR THE BURRITOS:

1 tablespoon unsalted butter

4 large eggs

2 tablespoons whole milk

¼ teaspoon kosher salt

⅛ teaspoon freshly ground black pepper

¼ cup shredded cheddar cheese

1 avocado, pitted, peeled, and mashed

4 (10-inch) plain or flavored flour tortillas, warmed

Roast the vegetables:

1. Preheat the oven to 425°F with a rack placed in the center of the oven. Line a sheet pan with parchment paper or aluminum foil.

2. Spread the vegetables on the prepared pan. Sprinkle the garlic on top, drizzle with the olive oil, and season with the herbes de Provence and a generous pinch each of salt and pepper. Use your hands to toss the vegetables, making sure they are evenly coated with the oil and seasonings.

3. Roast for 15 minutes, or until the vegetables are fork-tender.

Make the burritos:

4. While the vegetables are roasting, melt the butter in an 8- or 10-inch nonstick skillet over medium heat.

5. In a mixing bowl, whisk the eggs, milk, salt, and pepper. Pour the egg mixture into the skillet and use a rubber spatula to scrape the eggs as they begin to cook and curdle, working your way from the edges to the center. Continue pushing the curds around the pan until the eggs are fully scrambled and no longer runny. Stir in the cheese.

6. To assemble, spread a thin layer of mashed avocado in the center of a warm tortilla, followed by one-quarter each of the scrambled eggs and roasted vegetables. Fold the left and right edges of the tortilla and start to roll from the bottom up, tucking in the filling as you roll. Repeat with the remaining tortillas and fillings. Serve immediately.

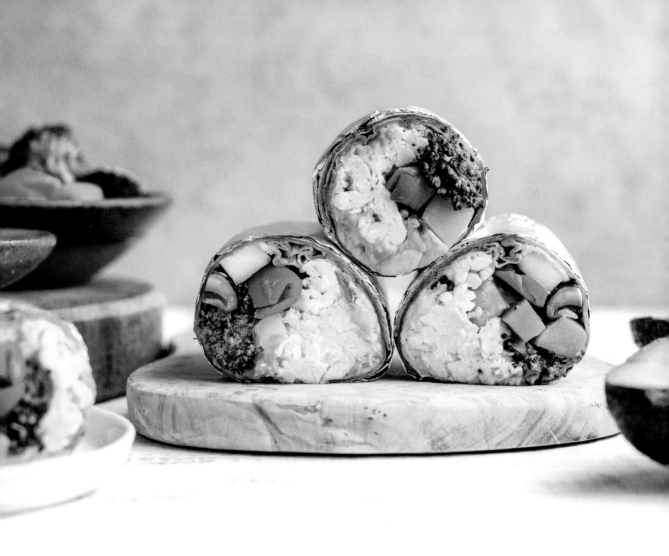

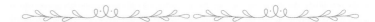

NOTES

When I can find them, I like to use spinach tortillas to give the burritos an extra veggie boost. If you can't find flavored tortillas, plain tortillas are just as delicious.

Fully assembled breakfast burritos can be wrapped in parchment paper and foil and stored in the refrigerator for up to 3 days or in the freezer for up to 3 months.

To reheat the burritos, remove the foil, place on a microwave-safe plate, and microwave for 1 to 2 minutes, or until heated through.

Corned Beef *and* Veggie Hash

Yield: 4 to 6 servings

Prep Time: 10 minutes

Cook Time: 25 minutes

When I was growing up, my dad was not exactly a cook, but he had a couple of dishes in his repertoire that he did well. I called it bachelor food, because that is what I imagined him cooking before he got married, and those were the dishes he would cook for us if my mom happened to be working an evening shift at the hospital. Many of the dishes were made with pantry staples, and a can of corned beef was always at the ready, just in case. It's been a long while since I opened a can of corned beef—now I prefer getting a high-quality marinated brisket from the butcher and cooking it at home—but I always make sure to set aside the leftovers for corned beef hash, just like my dad would make, but loaded with extra veggies!

2 tablespoons extra-virgin olive oil

1 cup finely chopped yellow onions (about 1 medium onion)

1 medium Yukon Gold potato, peeled and cut into ½-inch dice (about 1 cup)

½ teaspoon kosher salt

½ teaspoon paprika

2 cloves garlic, minced

¾ cup diced tomatoes

¼ cup diced red bell peppers

1 small sweet potato, peeled and cut into ½-inch dice (about 1 cup)

8 ounces leftover corned beef, shredded or chopped into ½-inch pieces

1 medium zucchini, cut into ½-inch dice (about 1 cup)

1 cup chopped kale

Freshly ground black pepper

1. Heat the olive oil in a large nonstick skillet over medium heat. Add the onions, potato, salt, and paprika and sauté until the potato is golden and nearly fork-tender, about 10 minutes.

2. Add the garlic and sauté for 30 seconds, then add the tomatoes, bell peppers, and sweet potato. Cook until the sweet potato is just about tender, another 7 to 10 minutes.

3. Stir in the corned beef, zucchini, and kale and cook until the zucchini is tender and the kale is wilted, about 5 minutes. Season to taste with additional salt and pepper. Serve immediately.

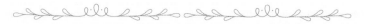

NOTES

Cooking the vegetables in stages results in veggies that are perfectly cooked with the perfect texture. I start with the longer-cooking vegetables (in this case, the potato) and end with the zucchini and kale, which need less time to cook. Tomatoes are the only exception; I add them earlier so they have plenty of time to break down.

If you find that the pan is drying out as you add the vegetables, you can add either a touch more olive oil or a splash of water or broth.

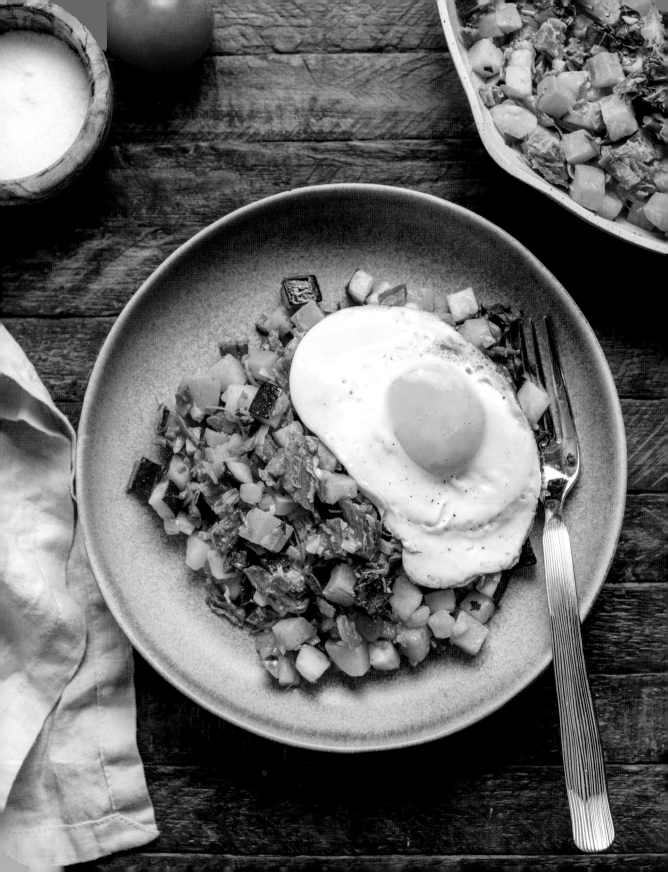

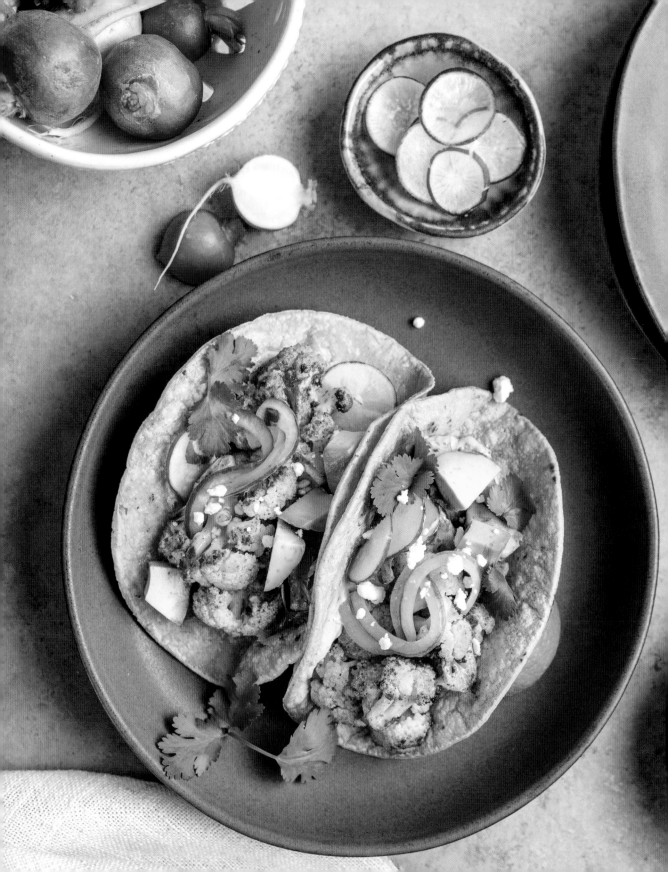

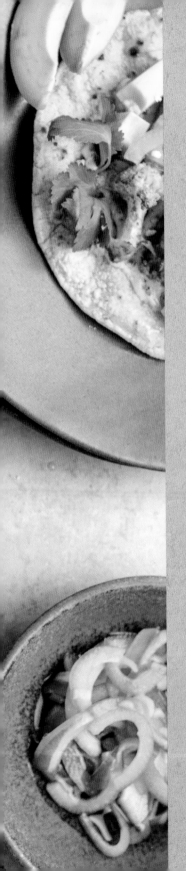

Appetizers and Small Plates

Yield: 4 to 6 servings

Prep Time: 40 minutes, plus 1 hour to rest dough

Cook Time: 20 minutes

Jackfruit Dumplings (Gyoza)

Dumplings are one of my family's favorite foods—I often keep gyoza prepped and ready in the freezer for simple lunches for my kids, and they're always a hit. These vegetable gyoza, made with a combination of jackfruit, cabbage, and mushrooms, are adapted from my mom's pork and cabbage gyoza, a recipe she inherited from one of her closest cousins, who married into a Japanese family and used to live part-time in Tokyo. If you've never cooked homemade dumplings, these gyoza are a great place to start!

FOR THE WRAPPERS:

2 cups all-purpose flour

½ teaspoon kosher salt

⅔ cup tepid water

FOR THE FILLING:

1 (14-ounce) can jackfruit (packed in brine), rinsed, drained, and minced

1 cup minced green cabbage

5 ounces oyster mushrooms, stems removed and minced

½ cup minced carrots

2 tablespoons minced green onions

2 teaspoons grated fresh ginger

1 tablespoon extra-virgin olive oil, for the pan

1 tablespoon plus 2 teaspoons soy sauce

1 teaspoon untoasted sesame oil (unrefined)

1 teaspoon oyster sauce

½ teaspoon granulated sugar

¼ teaspoon ground white pepper

1 to 2 tablespoons cornstarch

FOR THE DIPPING SAUCE:

¼ cup soy sauce

¼ cup rice wine vinegar

1 teaspoon hot chili oil (optional)

1 green onion, thinly sliced (optional)

4 tablespoons extra-virgin olive oil, divided, for the pan

1 cup boiling water, divided, for the pan

Make the wrapper dough:

1. In a food processor, combine the flour and salt. With the machine running, add the water in a thin stream until a loose ball forms.

2. Transfer the ball of dough to a lightly floured surface and knead for about 30 seconds. Wrap the dough in plastic wrap and let it rest for about 1 hour.

Make the filling:

3. In a large bowl, toss the jackfruit, cabbage, mushrooms, carrots, green onions, and ginger until combined.

4. Heat the olive oil in a medium skillet over medium heat. Add the jackfruit mixture and cook for 5 minutes, or until wilted. The mushrooms will have softened. Return the mixture to the bowl.

5. In a small bowl, whisk together the soy sauce, sesame oil, oyster sauce, sugar, and white pepper. Stir the mixture into the vegetables until they are evenly coated. Sprinkle 1 tablespoon of the cornstarch over the mixture and

(recipe continues on page 51)

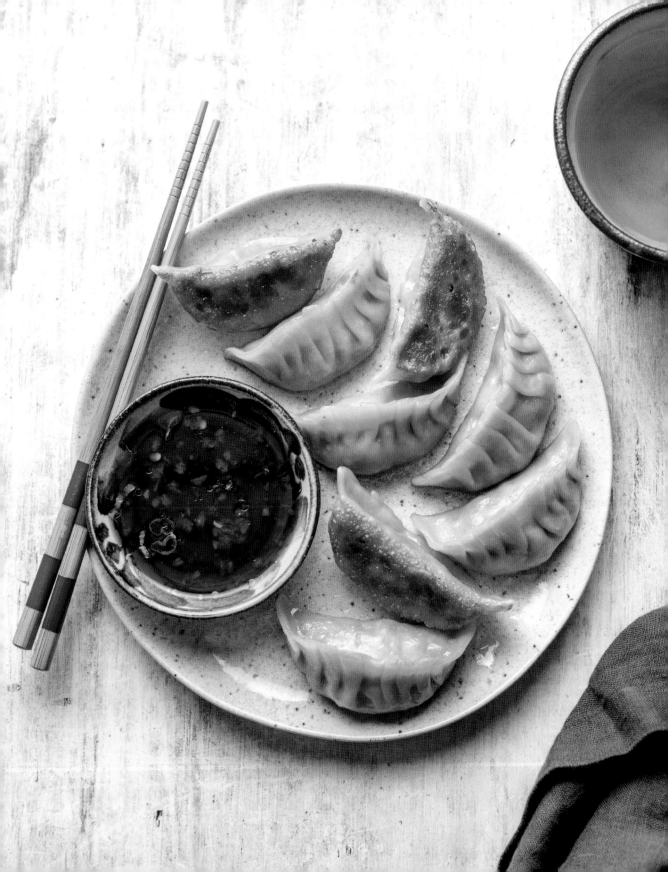

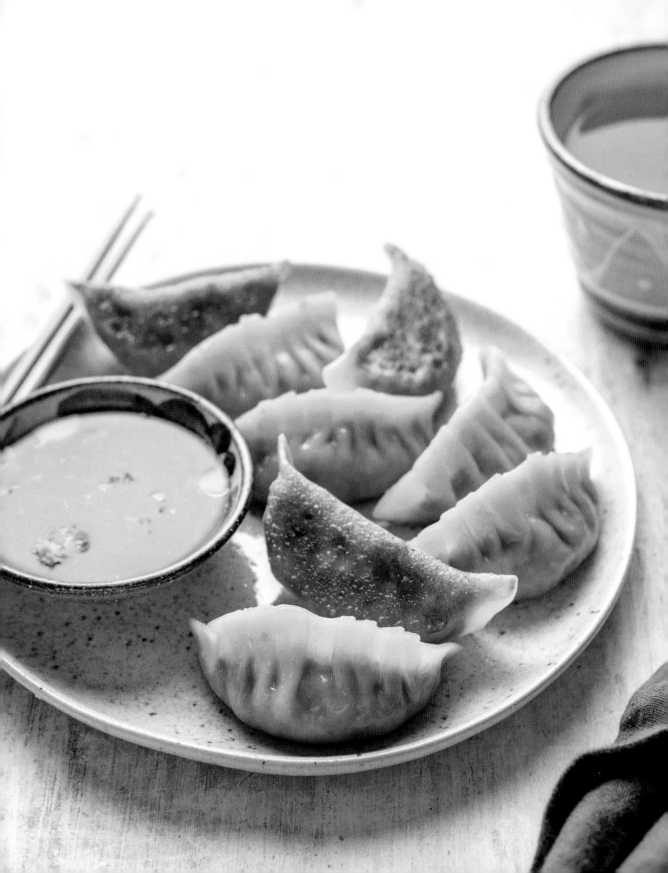

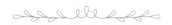

NOTES

Save time by using store-bought frozen gyoza wrappers, found at Asian grocers.

A food processor makes quick work of mincing and combining the ingredients for the filling.

Prepped gyoza keep well in the freezer; you can make batches of them, keep them in a freezer bag, and cook them from frozen. Add about 3 minutes to the overall cooking time.

Hot chili oil is a spicy condiment popular in Asian cooking and adds so much heat and flavor to the dipping sauce. The oil is infused with hot peppers, transforming it into a beautiful translucent red sauce speckled with chili flakes. You can find it in the Asian section of your local grocery store, at an Asian market, or even online. Lao Gan Ma Chili Crisp Sauce and Lee Kum Kee Chiu Chow Style Chili Oil are both good brands that are easy to find.

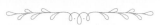

stir to combine. If the filling still seems too wet, mix in another tablespoon of cornstarch. Set the filling aside in the refrigerator while you make the dipping sauce and continue to work with the wrapper dough.

Make the dipping sauce:

6. In a small bowl, whisk together the soy sauce, vinegar, chili oil (if using), and green onion (if using). Set aside.

Assemble and cook the dumplings:

7. After the dough has rested for an hour, divide it in half. Wrap one half in plastic wrap and set it aside. Divide the remaining half into 12 equal pieces. Roll each piece on a lightly floured surface into a circle about 3 inches in diameter, with the center slightly thicker than the edges.

8. Place about 2 teaspoons of filling in the center of each wrapper. Fold in half, making a half-moon shape. Crimp to pleat the edges of the dough together, making a crescent shape. Set the completed dumplings on a lightly floured surface and cover loosely with wax paper.

9. Repeat with the other half of the dough and filling.

10. Heat a large nonstick skillet over medium heat. Pour in 2 tablespoons of the olive oil and, once hot, arrange half of the gyoza flat side down in the oil. Fry until the bottoms turn a light golden color, about 2 minutes. Pour ½ cup of the hot water into the pan, cover immediately, and cook for 5 minutes more. Drain the excess liquid. Pan-fry the gyoza until the bottoms are crisp and golden brown, about 3 minutes, adding a touch of oil if necessary to prevent them from sticking.

11. Repeat with the second batch of dumplings and the remaining olive oil and hot water.

12. Serve the gyoza immediately with the dipping sauce.

Yield: 4 servings
Prep Time: 10 minutes, plus 10 minutes to degorge zucchini
Cook Time: 20 minutes

Zucchini Fritters

When zucchini is in season, there's nothing easier than shredding it and transforming it into fritters! These fritters are baked rather than fried, and they are delicious with a dollop of sour cream or tzatziki. They are also a great side to salads or anything off the grill.

2 cups shredded zucchini (about 2 medium zucchini)

1½ teaspoons kosher salt, divided

1 large egg, beaten

⅓ cup grated Parmigiano-Reggiano cheese

¼ cup all-purpose flour

¼ cup panko breadcrumbs

1 clove garlic, minced

¼ cup finely chopped yellow onions

1½ teaspoons chopped fresh basil

Freshly ground black pepper

Tzatziki, homemade (page 76) or store-bought, or sour cream, for serving (optional)

Fresh herbs, such as flat-leaf parsley or mint, for garnish (optional)

1. Preheat the oven to 425°F with a rack placed in the center of the oven. Line a sheet pan with parchment paper and lightly brush the paper with olive oil.

2. Toss the zucchini with 1 teaspoon of the salt and place in a sieve set over a bowl for 10 minutes. Press the zucchini in the sieve, squeezing out the excess liquid.

3. Transfer the zucchini to a medium bowl and combine with the egg, cheese, flour, breadcrumbs, garlic, onions, and basil. Season with the remaining ½ teaspoon of salt and a pinch of pepper.

4. Using a small ice cream scoop or a large spoon, place a 2-tablespoon scoop on the prepared sheet pan. Lightly press until it is a disk, about ½ inch thick and 2½ inches in diameter. Repeat with the remaining zucchini mixture.

5. Bake for 10 minutes, then flip and bake for another 5 to 10 minutes, until the fritters are golden brown and cooked through. Serve with tzatziki or sour cream and garnish with herbs, If desired.

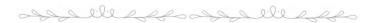

NOTE

The fritters can be reheated in a 375°F oven for 15 minutes. If you're in a rush, you can also microwave them in 40-second increments until warmed through.

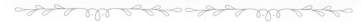

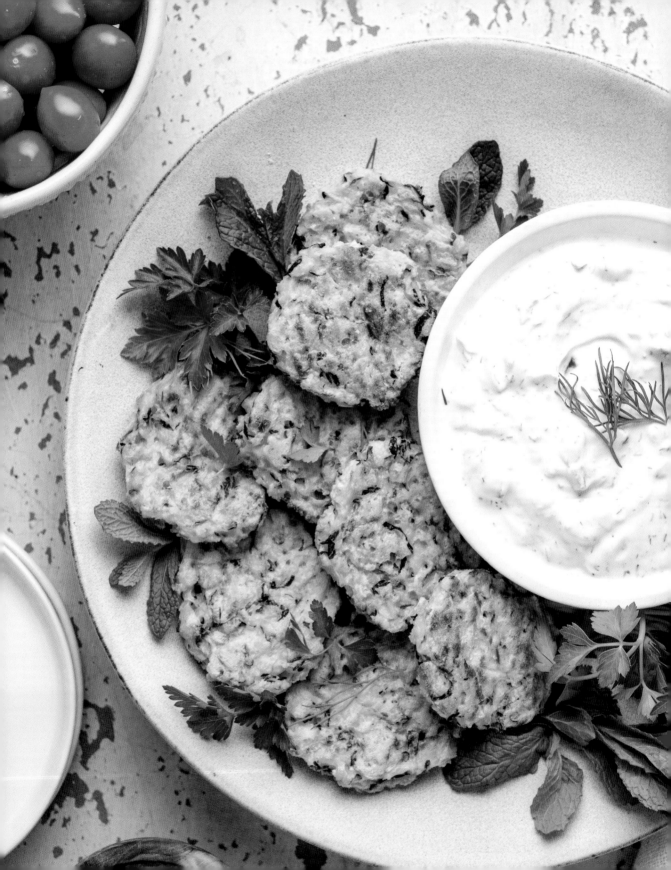

Sweet Potato Patties

Yield: 6 servings

Prep Time: 15 minutes

Cook Time: 25 minutes

If you love potato fritters, these sweet potato patties are for you! Full of fiber and antioxidants, they have the crunch of a fritter from the panko breadcrumb coating and are delicious served as an appetizer or with a salad.

1 large sweet potato (about 1¼ pounds)

1 tablespoon extra-virgin olive oil, plus more for frying

¼ cup finely diced onions

1 clove garlic, minced

¾ teaspoon Italian seasoning

1 cup panko breadcrumbs, divided

⅓ cup grated Parmigiano-Reggiano cheese

1 teaspoon kosher salt

⅛ teaspoon freshly ground black pepper

¼ cup all-purpose flour

1 large egg, beaten

⅓ cup crème fraîche or sour cream, for serving

Finely sliced fresh chives, for garnish

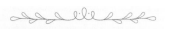

NOTE

The leftover sweet potato patties can be reheated in a 375°F oven for 15 minutes.

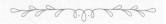

1. Pierce the sweet potato multiple times on all sides with a fork, then place on a microwave-safe plate and lightly tent with a damp paper towel. Microwave on high for 4 minutes, rotate, and continue to cook in 2-minute increments until it is soft. The exact cooking time will depend on your microwave's wattage. Let cool, then peel the sweet potato, place the flesh in a bowl, and use a fork to mash it.

2. In a 3-quart sauté pan, heat the olive oil over medium heat. Add the onions and sauté for about 4 minutes. Add the garlic and Italian seasoning and continue to sauté until the onions are translucent, another 3 minutes.

3. Place the onion mixture in the bowl with the mashed sweet potato and mix in ¼ cup of the breadcrumbs and the cheese. Season with the salt and pepper.

4. Using a standard-sized ice cream scoop, scoop a ball of the mixture, then use your hands to press it into a patty, about ½ inch thick and 3 inches in diameter. Repeat with the remaining mixture to make 6 patties.

5. Set up a breading station, putting the flour, egg, and remaining ¾ cup of breadcrumbs in three separate shallow bowls. Lightly dredge the patties in the flour, dip into the egg, and then into the breadcrumbs.

6. Heat about ¼ inch of olive oil in a large nonstick skillet over medium heat. Fry the sweet potato patties until golden brown, 4 to 5 minutes per side. Set on paper towels to drain. Serve with a dollop of crème fraîche or sour cream and a sprinkling of chives.

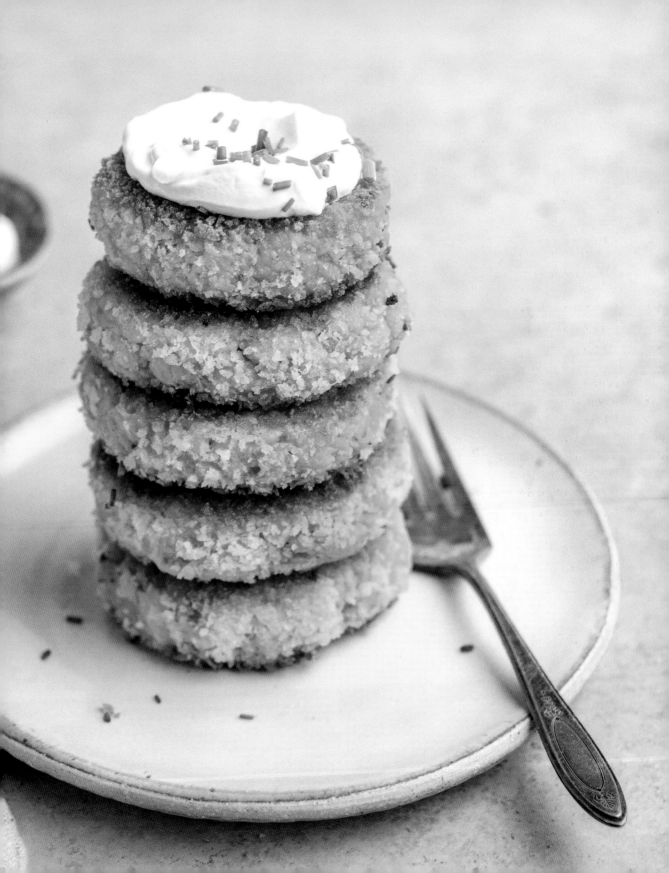

Yield: 4 to 6 servings

Prep Time: 15 minutes, plus 1 hour to rehydrate bulgur and 4 hours to rest meatball mixture

Cook Time: 1 hour 15 minutes

Mushroom Meatballs

When I think of the best meatballs I have ever eaten, the prize goes to my dear friend Rochelle. She uses a variety of ground meat in her meatballs, which are tender, flavorful, and simply the best. When I set out to create a meatless meatball, I had hers in mind as the gold standard. I like to think these mushroom meatballs are a close second when you want a meatless version, and my secret is bulgur! The grain adds a lovely texture and is the key to convincing any meat lover that meatballs can be made meatless.

¼ cup medium bulgur wheat

1 tablespoon extra-virgin olive oil

1 pound cremini or white mushrooms, finely chopped

½ cup finely chopped yellow onions

1 teaspoon soy sauce

1 teaspoon Worcestershire sauce

4 cloves garlic, minced

½ cup panko breadcrumbs

⅓ cup grated Parmigiano-Reggiano cheese, plus more for serving

½ teaspoon Italian seasoning

1 teaspoon chopped fresh flat-leaf parsley, plus more for garnish

2 large eggs, lightly beaten

Freshly ground black pepper

1 (24-ounce) jar marinara sauce

Toasted Italian bread, for serving

Prepare the meatball mixture:

1. Place the bulgur in a medium bowl, cover with boiling water, and let sit until the bulgur has absorbed the liquid and fluffed up. Depending on the fineness/coarseness of the grind, this can take anywhere from 15 minutes to 1 hour. It should yield about ½ cup of hydrated bulgur.

2. Heat the olive oil in a large skillet over medium-high heat. Add the mushrooms and onions, season with the soy sauce and Worcestershire sauce, and cook until the mushrooms have wilted and most of the liquid has cooked off, about 7 minutes. Stir in the garlic and cook for another 30 seconds. Transfer the mushroom mixture to a bowl and set aside.

3. Drain the bulgur thoroughly and add it to the bowl with the mushrooms. Mix in the breadcrumbs, cheese, Italian seasoning, parsley, eggs, and a few grinds of black pepper. Cover the bowl and place in the refrigerator to rest for at least 4 hours or overnight.

Cook the meatballs:

4. Preheat the oven to 400°F with a rack placed in the center of the oven. Line a sheet pan with parchment paper.

5. Using a small ice cream scoop or a large spoon, scoop 2-tablespoon portions of the mixture onto the prepared pan. Using your hands, roll each portion into a ball, pressing to compact it.

6. Bake for 15 minutes, or until the meatballs are firm to the touch.

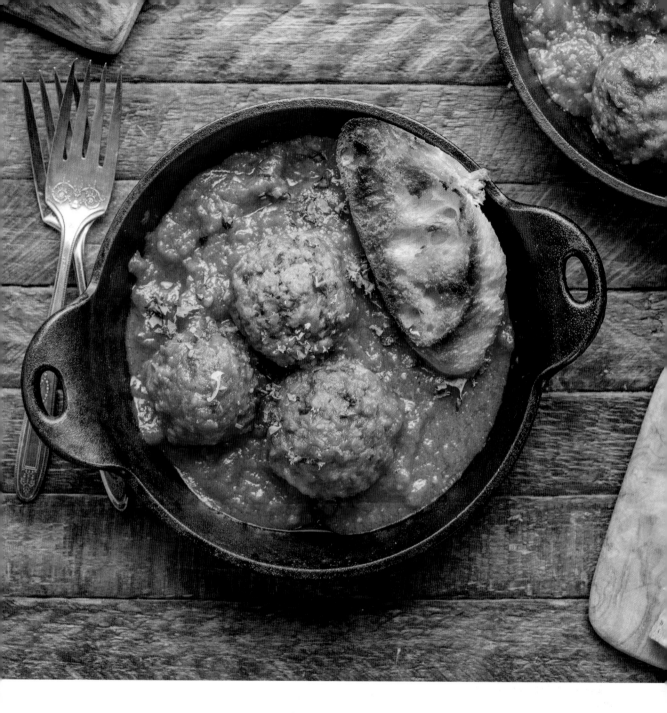

7. Bring the marinara sauce to a bubble in a large saucepan over medium heat. Transfer the meatballs to the sauce and lower the heat to a simmer. Cover and let the meatballs simmer in the sauce for 45 minutes.

8. Garnish the meatballs with chopped parsley and serve with toasted bread.

Pork *and* Beans Poutine

Yield: 4 servings

Prep Time: 10 minutes

Cook Time: 45 minutes

This recipe is an ode to my brother and father. When my brother went to university in Montreal, we were introduced to the wonders of poutine: salty fries smothered in gravy and cheese curds. I always thought they would be great with pork and beans, something my dad used to make for us when my mom was working a shift at the hospital. Not only does it work well; it's amazing!

FOR THE PORK AND BEANS:

2½ ounces thick-cut bacon, diced

⅓ cup diced yellow onions

3 tablespoons tomato sauce

2 tablespoons molasses

1 tablespoon apple cider vinegar

½ teaspoon Worcestershire sauce

½ teaspoon maple syrup

¼ teaspoon horseradish powder or wasabi powder

⅛ teaspoon freshly ground black pepper

⅛ teaspoon cayenne pepper

1 (15-ounce) can navy or cannellini beans

3 tablespoons cornstarch

2 tablespoons water

FOR THE STEAK FRIES:

1½ pounds potatoes (2 to 3 large potatoes), such as russet, Long White, or Yukon Gold, scrubbed

1 teaspoon kosher salt, divided

¼ cup extra-virgin olive oil

1 teaspoon paprika

¼ teaspoon cayenne pepper

¼ teaspoon garlic powder

1¼ cups crumbled cheese curds, for serving

Chopped fresh flat-leaf parsley, for garnish (optional)

Make the pork and beans:

1. Cook the bacon in a medium saucepan over medium heat for 3 to 5 minutes, or until the fat begins to render.

2. Add the onions to the pan and cook until translucent, about 7 minutes.

3. Stir in the tomato sauce, molasses, vinegar, Worcestershire sauce, maple syrup, horseradish powder, black pepper, and cayenne pepper, then add the beans with their canning liquid. Bring to a simmer and cook for about 15 minutes, stirring occasionally.

4. Stir together the cornstarch and water until smooth to make a slurry. Stir 1 tablespoon of the slurry into the bean mixture and allow to simmer for a few minutes, stirring often, until it thickens. If you want an even thicker sauce, add more of the slurry, 1 tablespoon at a time, keeping in mind that the sauce will thicken as it sits.

Make the fries:

5. Preheat the oven or an air fryer to 400°F.

6. Slice the potatoes in half lengthwise, then cut them into long wedges.

7. Place the potato wedges in a large saucepan and add enough water to cover them by about 1 inch. Stir in

(recipe continues on page 61)

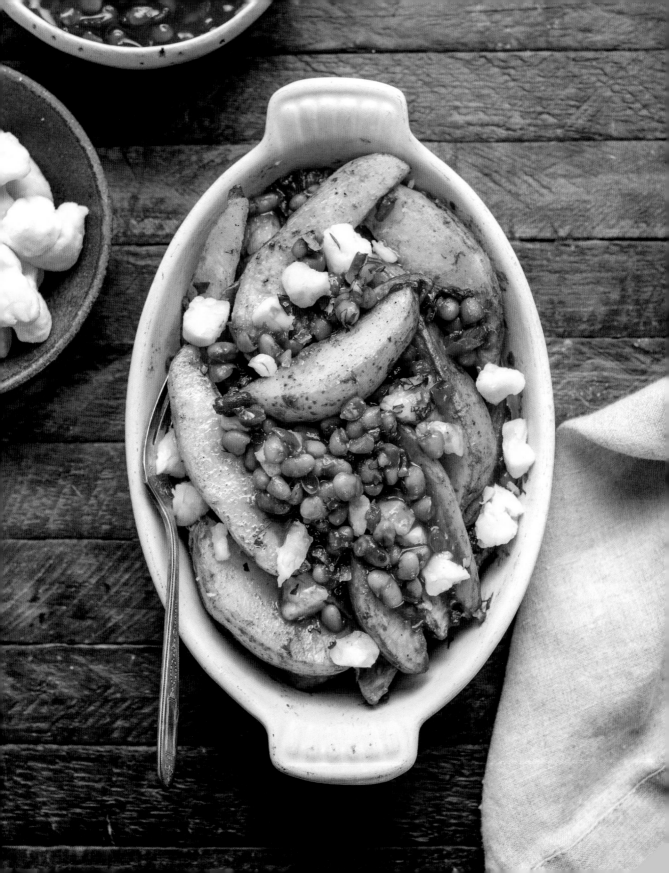

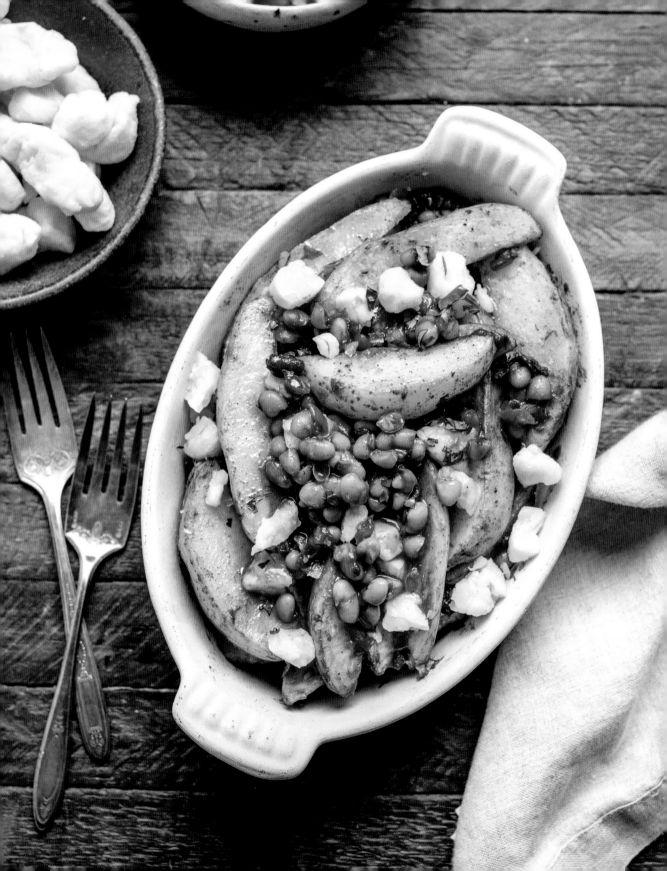

½ teaspoon of the salt. Bring to a boil and parboil the potatoes until the edges are tender but they are not fully fork-tender, 3 to 5 minutes.

8. Transfer the potato wedges to a tray covered with a clean dish towel or paper towels and pat them dry.

9. In a medium bowl, toss the potato wedges in the olive oil, coating them evenly. Sprinkle with the paprika, cayenne pepper, garlic powder, and remaining ½ teaspoon of salt, tossing to evenly coat the wedges in the seasonings. (After transferring the potatoes to the air fryer or oven, set the bowl aside; do not clean it.)

10. Air-fry the potato wedges for 15 minutes, or arrange the wedges on a sheet pan and bake for 15 to 20 minutes, until golden and crispy, flipping once halfway through. Return the fries to the bowl used to season the potatoes, tossing them in any residual olive oil left in the bowl, then transfer to a serving dish. Ladle the pork and beans over the fries, top with the cheese curds, and toss once more before serving. Garnish with parsley, if desired.

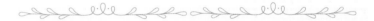

NOTES

The two components of this dish can be prepared simultaneously—while the beans simmer, you can easily prepare the fries, saving time. Also, you can make the beans a day or two in advance and reheat them before serving.

Cheese curds are created in the cheesemaking process—curds form when milk coagulates, and the whey is the liquid that is discarded when the curds are pressed to age into cheese. The curds can be eaten fresh; they are mild in flavor and satisfyingly squeaky to chew. Since curds are fresh and not aged, it can be tricky to source them in the US, which has strict laws regarding raw-milk cheeses. Some local cheesemakers and cheese mongers do sell cheese curds, but be sure to eat them as soon as possible because they lose their freshness quickly. If you can't find cheese curds, substitute torn mozzarella or diced Halloumi cheese.

Poutine is usually made with french fries, but I like to use steak fries in this version. The heartier fries have a broad surface, making it easier to scoop up the beans and curds. It also makes for a heartier, more satisfying appetizer!

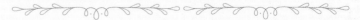

Stuffed Acorn Squash with Farro, Kale, and White Beans

Yield: 4 servings

Prep Time: 10 minutes

Cook Time: 40 minutes

When I was growing up, squash didn't exactly light me up the same way other vegetables could. Once I tried roasted squash, however, that was it—I was in love. Roasting acorn squash brings out its natural sweetness and makes it an ideal vessel for stuffing with all kinds of goodness. This stuffed acorn squash is made with sausage, but I also like making this dish completely meatless—it is great either way!

2 acorn squash

2 tablespoons extra-virgin olive oil, divided

1 teaspoon paprika

Kosher salt and freshly ground black pepper

8 ounces sweet Italian turkey or chicken sausage, casing removed

1 cup diced red onions (about 1 medium onion)

1 clove garlic, minced

1 cup canned white beans (any type), drained and rinsed

⅛ teaspoon cayenne pepper

1 teaspoon honey

1 cup cooked farro

2 cups chopped kale

1 tablespoon tomato paste

¼ cup crumbled feta cheese, plus more for serving

¼ cup roasted and salted shelled pumpkin seeds, for serving

1. Preheat the oven to 400°F with a rack placed in the lower third of the oven.

2. Slice the acorn squash in half lengthwise and remove the seeds. Scrape out a little well in each squash half to give the stuffing a place to settle. Place the halves cut side up in a baking dish. Brush the squash flesh with 1 tablespoon of the olive oil. Season with the paprika and sprinkle lightly with salt and pepper. Roast until the squash is tender and yields to a sharp knife, about 30 minutes.

3. Meanwhile, prepare the filling: Heat a large skillet over medium-high heat, then pour in the remaining tablespoon of olive oil. Add the sausage and cook until browned, crumbling it as it cooks, about 8 minutes, then stir in the onions and garlic and cook until the onions have wilted, about 3 minutes.

4. In a small bowl, toss the white beans with the cayenne pepper, honey, ¼ teaspoon of salt, and a little black pepper. Add the beans to the skillet and cook for 5 minutes. Stir in the farro, kale, and tomato paste and cook until the kale wilts, 3 to 5 minutes. Season to taste with salt and pepper. Remove from the heat.

5. When the squash is tender, remove it from the oven. Toss the feta cheese in the filling, then spoon it into the squash halves. Return the stuffed squash to the oven and roast until the stuffing is heated through, 5 to 7 minutes.

6. Top with the pumpkin seeds and additional feta cheese and serve.

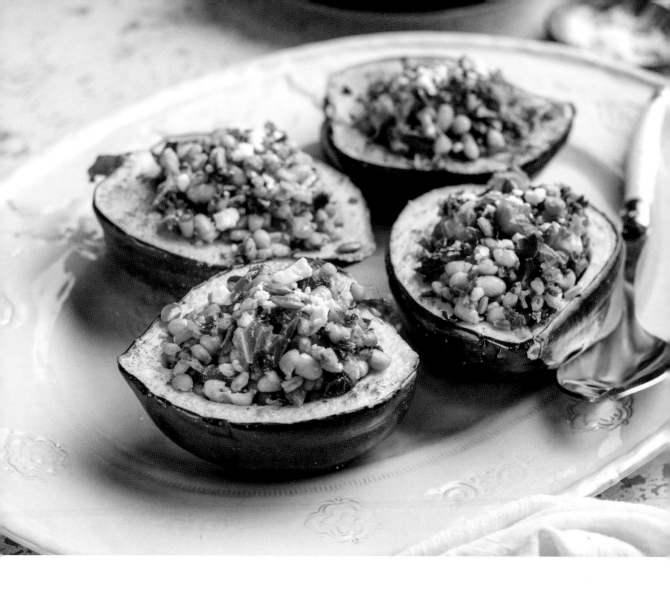

NOTE

Farro is a type of ancient grain, rich in protein and fiber, with a texture and appearance similar to barley. Popular in Italy, farro is now easily found here in the US, and it is perfect for bowls, as an alternative to rice, or in dishes like this one. I keep a bag of quick-cooking farro in the pantry and love to make a batch to enjoy throughout the week, throwing it in salads or soups, or eating it as a simple side. In general, 1 cup of dry farro makes 2 cups of cooked farro, so for this recipe, if you don't have any leftover farro, you can make 1 cup of cooked farro from ½ cup of dry.

Shrimp *and* Cauliflower Grits

Yield: 4 to 6 servings
Prep Time: 10 minutes
Cook Time: 15 minutes

I can never resist creamy, cheesy grits, but I think of it as a once-a-year kind of meal. Making cauliflower grits fixes that—these "grits" are just as delicious and made for enjoying more than once a year for sure.

FOR THE CAULIFLOWER GRITS:

1 large head cauliflower

½ cup chicken stock

½ cup whole milk

3 tablespoons unsalted butter

½ cup shredded aged white cheddar cheese

Kosher salt and freshly ground black pepper

FOR THE SHRIMP:

1 tablespoon extra-virgin olive oil

1 clove garlic, minced

2 teaspoons creole seasoning

1 pound extra-large shrimp, peeled and deveined

Kosher salt and freshly ground black pepper

¼ cup white wine

2 tablespoons unsalted butter

Minced fresh flat-leaf parsley, for garnish

1. Trim and discard the leaves and tough base of the cauliflower stalk. Cut the florets off the stalk and set aside. Peel the stalk, then roughly chop it into 1-inch chunks.

2. Place the chopped cauliflower stalk in a food processor. Pulse until chopped, then add the florets and continue to pulse until the cauliflower has a texture reminiscent of rice.

3. Transfer the cauliflower rice to a medium saucepan. Add the chicken stock, milk, and butter and bring to a simmer over medium heat. Cook the cauliflower, stirring occasionally, until it thickens to the consistency of grits, about 10 minutes.

4. Meanwhile, cook the shrimp: Heat the olive oil in a sauté pan over medium-low heat. Add the garlic and cook for 30 seconds. Stir in the creole seasoning and cook for another 30 seconds, then add the shrimp and a pinch each of salt and pepper, stirring well. Deglaze the pan with the wine, then stir in the butter. Cook for a few minutes more, until the shrimp have curled slightly and are opaque.

5. Finish the grits by stirring in the cheese and seasoning with salt and pepper to taste.

6. To serve, spoon the grits into bowls and top with the shrimp and sauce. Garnish with parsley and serve immediately.

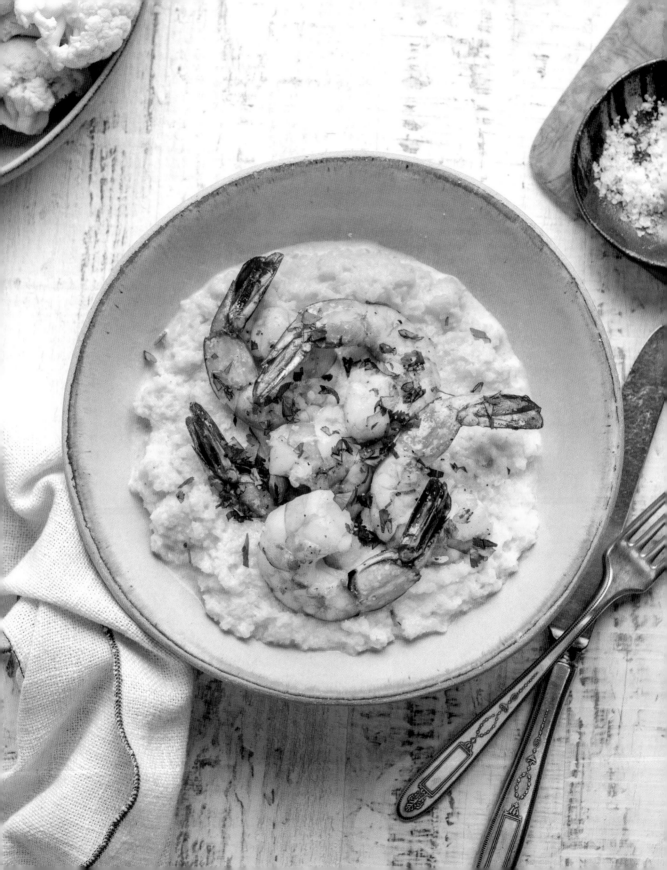

Stuffed Portobello Mushrooms *and* Spicy Romesco Sauce

Yield: 8 servings

Prep Time: 20 minutes

Cook Time: 45 minutes

I'll never forget encountering my first mushroom hater. I couldn't even imagine it was possible, but I soon learned that mushroom hate is a textural thing. I've always adored mushrooms and how versatile they are, especially for adding a meaty texture to dishes, so imagine my surprise when my son confessed to me that he hates mushrooms! I have made it my goal to find a recipe that could convince mushroom haters to reconsider. These stuffed mushrooms might do the trick! The magical ingredient is the spicy romesco sauce, which adds a nutty, hearty punch to each bite. Even if it doesn't convert everyone to mushrooms, I can take comfort in knowing that at least my husband has declared this one of his favorite recipes in this book. As for my son, well, I'm still working on him!

FOR THE MUSHROOMS:

8 large portobello mushrooms, stems removed

2 tablespoons extra-virgin olive oil

Kosher salt and freshly ground black pepper

FOR THE ROMESCO SAUCE:

½ cup chopped toasted hazelnuts

¼ cup diced tomatoes

1 roasted red pepper (jarred is fine)

1 clove garlic, chopped

1 tablespoon tomato paste

1 tablespoon red wine or sherry vinegar

1½ teaspoons paprika

½ teaspoon cayenne pepper

½ teaspoon kosher salt

¼ cup extra-virgin olive oil

FOR THE STUFFING:

2 tablespoons extra-virgin olive oil, divided

4 cups chopped kale

2 cups cauliflower rice

Kosher salt and freshly ground black pepper

½ cup shredded mozzarella cheese, or 8 thin slices fresh mozzarella

¼ cup panko breadcrumbs

Roast the mushrooms:

1. Preheat the oven to 425°F with a rack placed in the center of the oven. Have a sheet pan on hand; for best results, line it with an ovenproof wire cooling rack (see Notes).

2. Place the mushrooms on the sheet pan with the gills facing up. Brush the gills with the olive oil and season lightly with salt and pepper.

3. Roast the mushrooms for 15 to 20 minutes, or until they have begun to soften and release their juices.

Make the romesco sauce:

4. Meanwhile, place the hazelnuts, diced tomatoes, roasted red pepper, garlic, tomato paste, vinegar, paprika, cayenne pepper, and salt in a small food processor and purée until smooth. With the machine running, slowly pour in the olive oil and process until smooth.

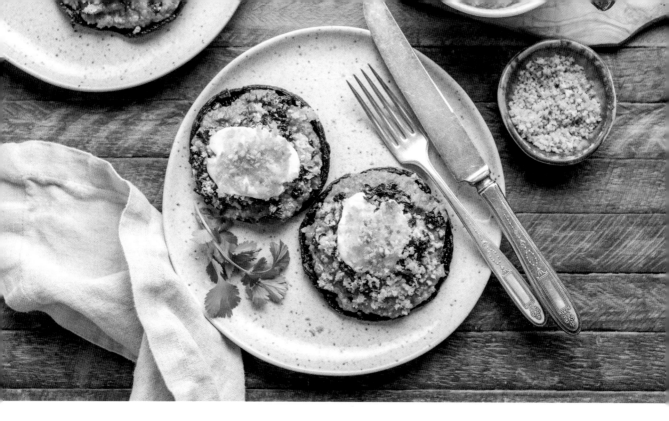

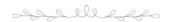

NOTES

I line my sheet pan with an ovenproof wire cooling rack, which allows air to circulate around the mushrooms and any juices that are released to drain. If you don't have an ovenproof rack, take extra care to discard any liquid.

I keep store-bought riced cauliflower in the freezer—it's perfect for throwing into dishes like this one!

Preshredded mozzarella is a refrigerator staple for recipes like this, but when I have fresh mozzarella, I sometimes opt for it instead, placing thin slices on top of the mushrooms as shown above.

Make the stuffing and mushrooms:

5. Heat 1 tablespoon of the olive oil in a large skillet over medium heat. Add the kale and cauliflower rice and season lightly with salt and pepper. Cook until the kale has wilted, about 3 minutes. Set aside.

6. When the mushrooms have softened, remove them from the oven and discard any liquid they have released. Return them to the sheet pan, cap side down. Fill each mushroom with romesco sauce, then top with the kale and cauliflower mixture and mozzarella. Season lightly with pepper.

7. Mix the breadcrumbs with the remaining tablespoon of olive oil and sprinkle on top of the mushrooms.

8. Bake the stuffed mushrooms for 15 to 20 minutes, or until the centers are tender. Thicker, meatier mushrooms may take more time to cook; lightly tent the mushrooms with aluminum foil if you find that the breadcrumbs are golden brown before the mushrooms are fully tender.

9. Serve immediately.

Steak Fries *with* Chimichurri

Yield: 4 servings
Prep Time: 10 minutes
Cook Time: 30 minutes

Confession time: while fries are usually enjoyed as a side dish or appetizer, I can make a meal out of them. Steak fries are my weakness, and so is a tangy, herby chimichurri. Put them together and the plate won't last long!

FOR THE STEAK FRIES:

3 to 4 medium potatoes, such as russet, Long White, or Yukon Gold, scrubbed, sliced in half lengthwise, and then cut into wedges

1 teaspoon kosher salt, divided

¼ cup extra-virgin olive oil

1 teaspoon paprika

¼ teaspoon cayenne pepper

¼ teaspoon garlic powder

FOR THE CHIMICHURRI:

3 large cloves garlic, smashed with the side of a knife

2½ cups fresh cilantro leaves

¼ cup sherry vinegar

⅓ cup extra-virgin olive oil

1 teaspoon kosher salt

¼ teaspoon cayenne pepper

1. Preheat the oven or an air fryer to 400°F.

   Place the potato wedges in a large saucepan and add enough water to cover them by about 1 inch. Stir in ½ teaspoon of the salt. Bring to a boil and parboil the potatoes until the edges are tender but the potatoes are not fully fork-tender, 3 to 5 minutes.

2. Transfer the potatoes to a tray covered with a clean dish towel or paper towels and pat them dry.

3. In a medium bowl, toss the potato wedges in the olive oil, coating them evenly. Season with the paprika, cayenne pepper, garlic powder, and remaining ½ teaspoon of salt, tossing to evenly coat the wedges in the spices and salt. (After transferring the fries to the air fryer or oven, set the bowl aside; do not clean it.)

4. Air-fry the fries for 15 minutes, or arrange the fries on a sheet pan and bake for 15 to 20 minutes, until golden and crispy, flipping once halfway through.

5. Meanwhile, make the chimichurri: Using a food processor, finely chop the garlic. Add the cilantro, vinegar, olive oil, salt, and cayenne pepper and pulse until the cilantro is finely chopped. Set aside.

6. When the fries are done, return them to the bowl used to season the potatoes, tossing them in any residual olive oil left in the bowl, then transfer to a serving dish. Serve immediately with the chimichurri.

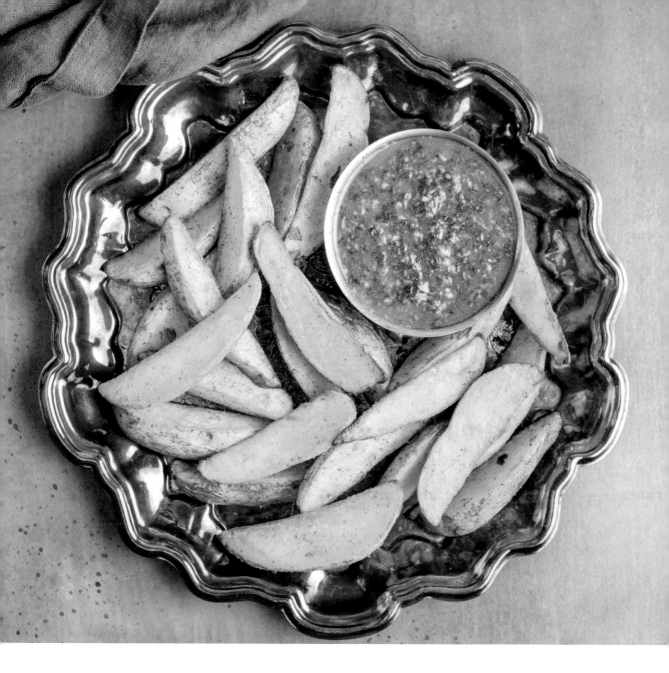

NOTE

The chimichurri can be made up to 48 hours in advance but is best if used within 24 hours. Store it in an airtight glass container in the refrigerator until ready to use. Let it come to room temperature before serving.

Veggie Nachos

Yield: 6 servings
Prep Time: 15 minutes
Cook Time: 10 minutes

I don't make nachos often, but when I do, I make sure they're loaded with so much goodness that they are practically a meal. My husband and I have been known to chow down on a whole tray by ourselves while watching a movie. Once you try these nachos, you'll soon understand why!

FOR THE AVOCADO-CILANTRO SAUCE:

2 cloves garlic, peeled

1 teaspoon kosher salt

½ cup sour cream

1 ripe avocado, pitted and peeled

¼ cup fresh cilantro leaves

Juice of ½ lime

Freshly ground black pepper

FOR THE NACHOS:

10 ounces thick tortilla chips

1 (15-ounce) can pinto beans, drained and rinsed

2 cups shredded cheddar cheese

1 cup chopped or sliced vegetables of choice (corn, bell pepper, mushrooms, etc.)

½ cup crumbled Cotija or feta cheese, plus more for topping

⅓ cup sliced black olives

¼ cup pickled jalapeños

½ cup salsa

¼ cup Quick-Pickled Red Onions (opposite)

¼ cup finely diced red onions

¼ cup thinly sliced radishes

¼ cup sliced green onions

¼ cup chopped fresh cilantro

1. Preheat the oven to 400°F with a rack placed in the center of the oven.

Make the sauce:

2. In a small food processor, process the garlic and salt until finely chopped. Add the sour cream, avocado, cilantro, lime juice, and a few grinds of pepper. Blend until smooth. Adjust the seasoning with salt and pepper if necessary. The sauce can be prepared ahead of time and stored in a tightly sealed container in the refrigerator for up to 3 days.

Make the nachos:

3. Line a sheet pan with parchment paper and spread the tortilla chips in an even layer, lightly overlapping the chips so there aren't any gaps.

4. Spread the pinto beans evenly over the chips, followed by the cheddar cheese, vegetables, Cotija cheese, black olives, and pickled jalapeños. Bake for about 10 minutes, until the cheese is melted.

5. Remove the nachos from the oven and top with the avocado-cilantro sauce, salsa, pickled onions, red onions, radishes, green onions, cilantro, and a little more Cotija cheese. Serve hot.

Quick-Pickled Red Onions

Yield: 2 cups (6 to 8 servings)

Prep Time: 5 minutes, plus 30 minutes to pickle

Cook Time: 5 minutes

I love keeping a batch of quick-pickled onions handy to add extra pop to any dish. Use them in Veggie Nachos (opposite), Spicy Cauliflower Tacos (page 72), and more!

¾ cup distilled white vinegar

¼ cup water

2 tablespoons granulated sugar

1½ teaspoons kosher salt

1 medium red onion, thinly sliced

1. In a small bowl, stir together the vinegar, water, sugar, and salt until the sugar and salt have dissolved.

2. Place the sliced onion in a jar. Pour the vinegar mixture over the onion and let sit at room temperature for at least 30 minutes, but preferably for 1 hour.

3. Serve immediately or keep refrigerated for future use. The onions will keep for up to 2 weeks.

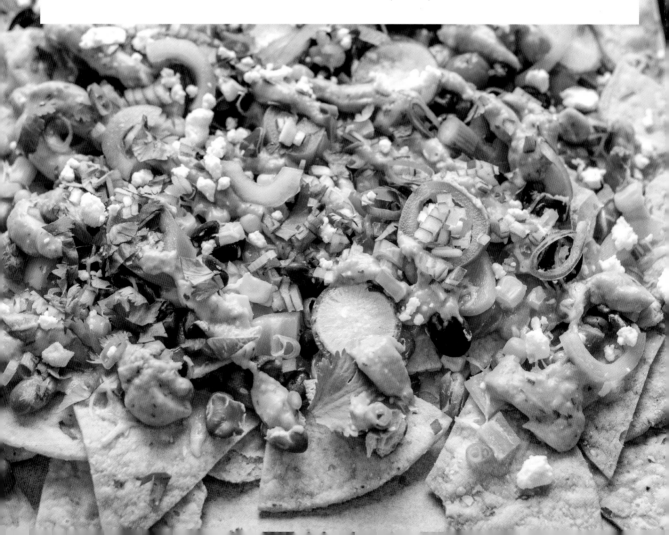

Spicy Cauliflower Tacos

Yield: 4 servings
Prep Time: 10 minutes
Cook Time: 35 minutes

Cauliflower is like a chameleon—it adapts well to its environment. While it doesn't change color, it takes on flavors with ease. I just love using roasted cauliflower in these spicy tacos! The sauce gives it that extra kick, perfect for spicing up taco night.

FOR THE CAULIFLOWER:

1 large head cauliflower, cut into bite-sized florets

¼ cup extra-virgin olive oil

2 teaspoons ground cumin

2 teaspoons smoked paprika

1 teaspoon ground coriander

¼ teaspoon cayenne pepper

Kosher salt

FOR THE SAUCE:

½ cup sour cream

½ chipotle pepper in adobo sauce

1 clove garlic, minced

2 tablespoons lime juice

FOR SERVING:

12 (4½-inch) corn tortillas

¼ cup Quick-Pickled Red Onions (page 71)

1 avocado, pitted, peeled, and diced

½ cup thinly sliced radishes

½ cup crumbled Cotija cheese or feta cheese

Fresh cilantro leaves, for garnish

Lime wedges, for serving

1. Preheat the oven to 450°F with a rack placed in the center of the oven.

2. In a bowl, toss the cauliflower florets with the olive oil until they are evenly coated on all sides. Season with the cumin, paprika, coriander, cayenne pepper, and a generous sprinkling of salt and toss to evenly coat.

3. Scatter the cauliflower on a sheet pan and roast for 20 to 35 minutes, or until browned on all sides and fork-tender, tossing the cauliflower halfway through cooking.

4. While the cauliflower roasts, make the sauce: Place the sour cream, chipotle pepper, garlic, and lime juice in a small food processor. Process until smooth, then set aside.

5. When ready to serve, warm the tortillas in a skillet over medium heat. Spread a little sauce on each tortilla and top with the cauliflower, pickled onions, avocado, radishes, cheese, and cilantro. Serve with lime wedges.

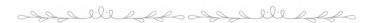

NOTE

Chipotle peppers can be very spicy. If you prefer a milder sauce, start with half a pepper and build to taste. Or, if you're very sensitive to spice, use just a few drops of the creamy chipotle sauce.

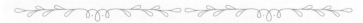

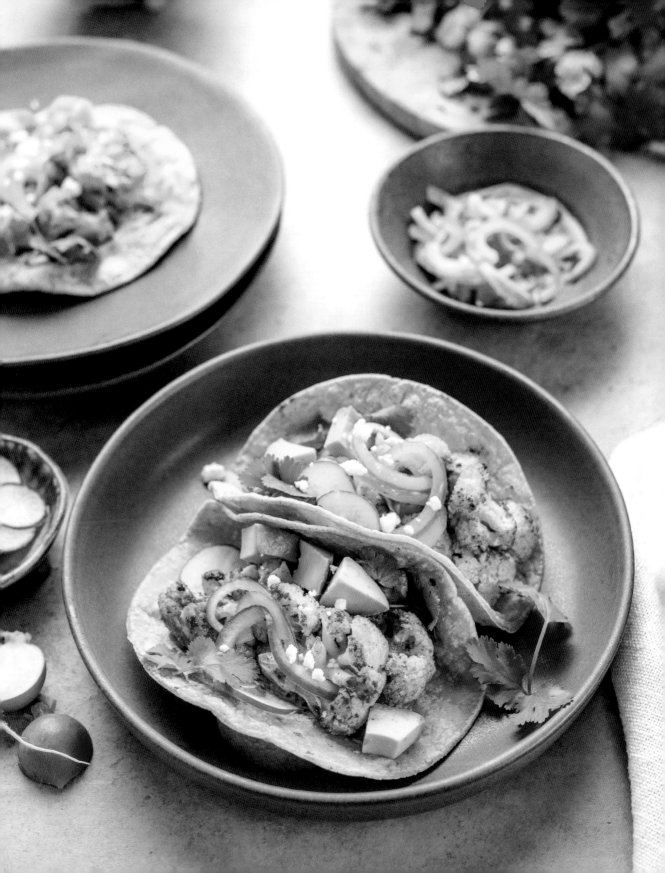

Buffalo Cauliflower "Wings"

Yield: 4 servings

Prep Time: 10 minutes

Cook Time: 45 minutes

When I think of wings, I can't help but think of my freshman year of college, when I thought nothing of eating wings and a pint of ice cream after a night of studying. I quickly learned that wasn't a wise or sustainable way to eat, but imagine if I'd known about cauliflower wings back then? These wings are much better for you and still give you that spicy kick you crave!

1 cup buttermilk

⅔ cup all-purpose flour

½ teaspoon salt

¼ teaspoon cayenne pepper

¼ teaspoon ground coriander

¼ teaspoon ground cumin

¼ teaspoon paprika

1 head cauliflower, cut into bite-sized florets

2 cups panko breadcrumbs

½ cup Buffalo sauce, divided

Ranch or blue cheese dressing, for serving

Celery sticks, for serving

Thinly sliced green onions, for garnish (optional)

1. Preheat the oven to 450°F with a rack placed in the center of the oven. Line a sheet pan with parchment paper.

2. In a large bowl, whisk together the buttermilk, flour, salt, cayenne pepper, coriander, cumin, and paprika until smooth.

3. Add the cauliflower florets to the batter and use a large spoon to toss the florets until evenly coated.

4. Place the breadcrumbs in a separate bowl. Use a spider strainer or a slotted spoon to transfer the florets into the breadcrumbs to lightly coat. Spread out the breaded florets on the prepared pan, spacing them evenly.

5. Bake for 20 minutes, then transfer to a large bowl along with ¼ cup of the Buffalo sauce. Toss to coat the florets well. Return the coated florets to the pan and bake for another 20 to 25 minutes, until the breading is crispy and the cauliflower is tender.

6. Serve immediately with the remaining ¼ cup of Buffalo sauce, ranch or blue cheese dressing, and celery sticks. Garnish with sliced green onions, if desired.

NOTE

Cauliflower wings are best enjoyed immediately, but if you have any leftovers, you can reheat them in a 375°F oven for about 10 minutes, until heated through.

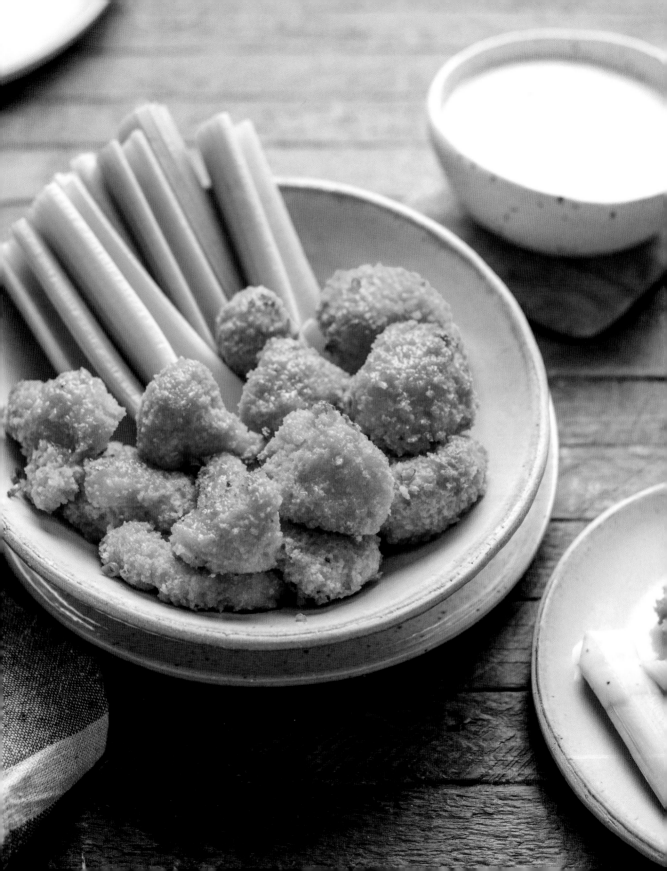

Yield: 2¼ cups (16 servings)

Prep Time: 5 minutes, plus 2 hours 15 minutes to drain and chill

Tzatziki

Tzatziki is one of those sauces I always keep on hand in the refrigerator. It's perfect served as a dip with fresh crudités, adding brightness to crunchy vegetables. But it is a wonderful addition to many other dishes. It's a must on my Gyro Flatbread (page 90), and it's delicious with the Zucchini Fritters on page 52, on top of the Mushroom Burgers on page 82, drizzled on the Falafel Bowls on page 164, and more! If you don't want to make your own, it's easy to find good-quality store-bought tzatziki these days (Boar's Head makes an excellent one, for example). But my recipe is simple and easy to prepare.

1 (17-ounce) container plain Greek yogurt (see Notes)

1 medium cucumber, quartered lengthwise and thinly sliced

1 tablespoon extra-virgin olive oil, plus more for drizzling if desired

4 cloves garlic, minced

1 teaspoon kosher salt

2 teaspoons sherry vinegar

1 tablespoon chopped fresh dill, plus extra for garnish if desired

1. Place the yogurt in a clean cheesecloth or tea towel, gather up the edges, and suspend it over a bowl in the refrigerator for 2 hours. After 2 hours, squeeze out the excess liquid.

2. Place the cucumber slices in another cheesecloth and gently squeeze out any liquid.

3. Combine the strained yogurt, cucumber slices, olive oil, garlic, salt, vinegar, and dill in a bowl and refrigerate for at least 15 minutes before using. Garnish with a drizzle of olive oil and/or a sprinkling of fresh dill, if desired.

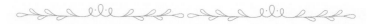

NOTES

Store the tzatziki in an airtight container in the refrigerator for up to 3 days.

Since the yogurt is the shining star in tzatziki, use the best plain Greek yogurt you can find. I recommend Fage—it's a high-quality, creamy yogurt that can easily be found at most grocers. Depending on the brand you use, the yogurt may need less straining time or, in some cases, no straining at all; for example, Fage is so thick that I often skip the straining altogether, which saves me time when I want tzatziki in a hurry.

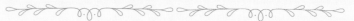

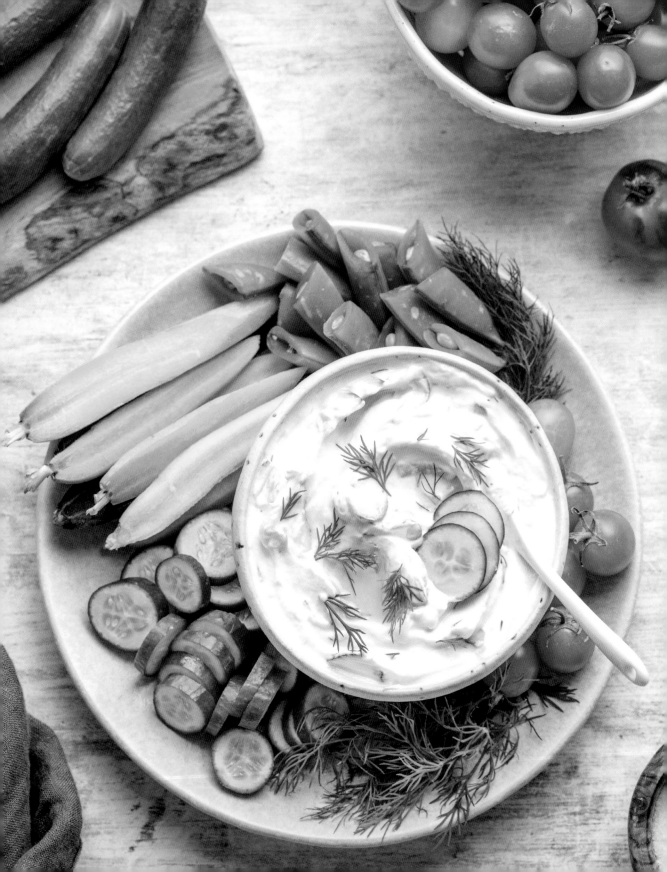

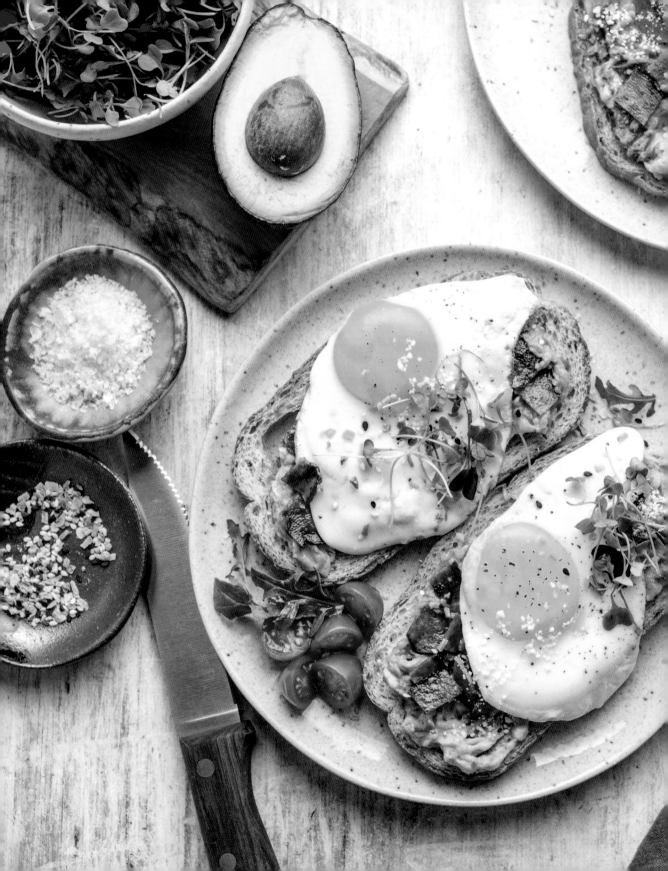

Sandwiches, Flatbreads, and Burgers

Ratatouille Sandwiches *with* Chicken Sausage

Yield: 4 servings

Prep Time: 10 minutes

Cook Time: 40 minutes

I've always loved sausage and pepper sandwiches, but I often felt there was something missing. This version takes inspiration from a classic ratatouille, with summer squash and eggplant joining forces with peppers and onions for my idea of the ideal sandwich, loaded with all the summer veggies!

4 links chicken sausage, hot Italian style

½ cup water

4 tablespoons extra-virgin olive oil, divided

1 medium eggplant, cut into ½-inch cubes

Kosher salt

1 cup diced red onions (about 1 medium onion)

4 cloves garlic, minced

1 red bell pepper, chopped into ½-inch pieces

1 orange bell pepper, chopped into ½-inch pieces

1 (14.5-ounce) can diced tomatoes

2 tablespoons tomato paste

1 teaspoon herbes de Provence

2 zucchini, chopped into 1-inch pieces

1 teaspoon sherry vinegar

2 tablespoons chopped fresh basil

4 sausage/brat buns, toasted, for serving

1 tablespoon chopped fresh flat-leaf parsley, for garnish

1. Place the sausage links in a skillet with the water. Cook over medium heat for 10 minutes, turning periodically, until the water has evaporated and the sausages are browned on all sides. Set aside.

2. Meanwhile, begin making the ratatouille: Heat 2 tablespoons of the olive oil in a sauté pan over medium heat. Add the eggplant and a pinch of salt and cook, stirring often, until the eggplant has softened and is lightly browned on all sides, about 8 minutes. Transfer to a plate and set aside.

3. Add the remaining 2 tablespoons of oil to the pan with the onions and garlic. Cook until the onions have softened and are translucent, about 4 minutes. Stir in the bell peppers and cook until the peppers have softened, another 4 minutes. Stir in the diced tomatoes, tomato paste, and herbes de Provence and bring to a boil. Lower the heat, cover, and simmer, stirring occasionally, until the tomatoes have broken down and the sauce is flavorful, 15 to 20 minutes.

4. Slice the sausages into 1-inch chunks and add to the pan along with the zucchini and cooked eggplant. Cook until the zucchini is fork-tender, about 5 minutes.

5. Stir in the vinegar and adjust the seasoning as necessary with salt and pepper. Stir in the basil and turn off the heat.

6. To serve, nestle the sausage and vegetables in the toasted buns and garnish with the parsley.

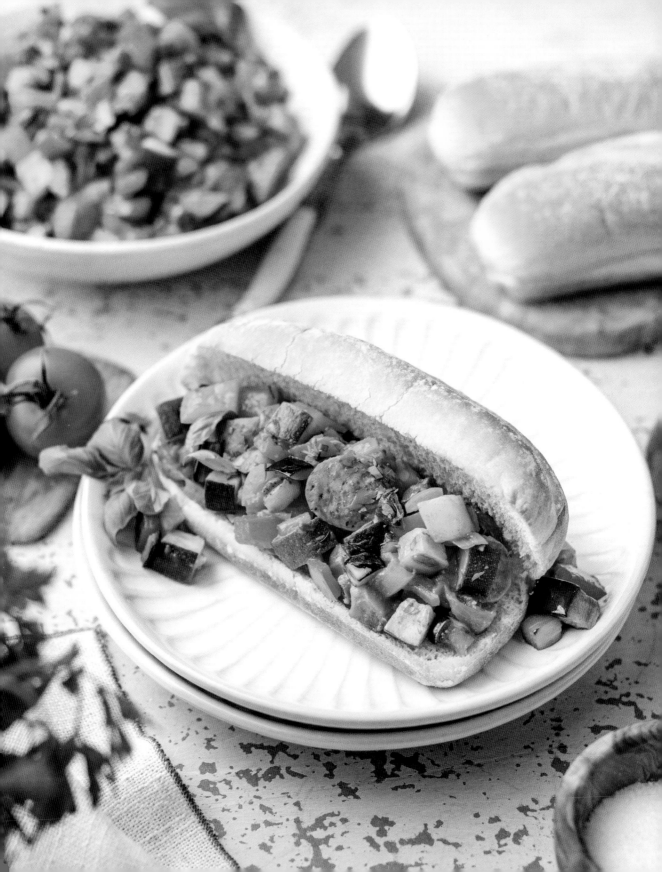

Yield: 4 servings

Prep Time: 5 minutes, plus 15 minutes to marinate

Cook Time: 8 minutes

Mushroom Burgers

The first time I had a mushroom burger, I thought, "Who needs meat?" Even though I still love a meaty burger once in a while, mushroom burgers are something I can eat all the time! A simple marinade makes them juicy and flavorful.

4 portobello mushrooms

3 tablespoons extra-virgin olive oil

2 tablespoons balsamic vinegar

2 cloves garlic, minced

Kosher salt and freshly ground black pepper

4 hamburger buns, toasted, for serving

SUGGESTED TOPPINGS:

Mayonnaise and/or other condiments of choice

Tomato slices

Lettuce leaves

Onion slices

1. Wipe the mushrooms clean and remove the stems. Drizzle the olive oil over the mushroom caps and use your fingers or a pastry brush to evenly coat them on all sides with the oil. Do the same with the vinegar. Turn the mushrooms stem side up and sprinkle with the garlic and a generous pinch each of salt and pepper. Let the mushrooms marinate for 10 to 15 minutes.

2. Preheat a grill to medium-high heat, or heat a grill pan or heavy pan, such as a cast-iron skillet, over medium-high heat. Grill or cook the mushrooms until the centers are tender, 3 to 4 minutes per side.

3. Serve the mushroom burgers on the toasted buns with your favorite toppings.

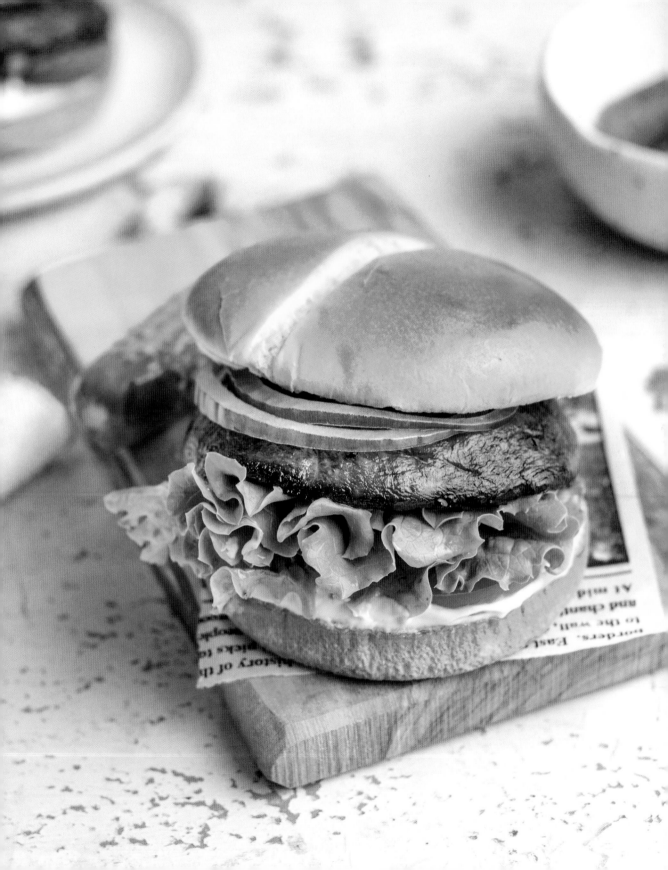

Yield: 4 servings

Prep Time: 10 minutes, plus 20 minutes to pickle veggies

Cook Time: 8 minutes

Spiced Potato Wraps

Here in the Bay Area, there is a restaurant that makes my favorite Bombay potato dosa wraps. The spiced potatoes are wrapped in paper-thin dosas (south Indian pancakes/crepes) and served with pickled carrots and radishes—it's one of my favorite lunches when I'm out and about. In this homemade version, I use flour tortillas in place of dosas for the wraps and fill them with fragrant spiced potatoes and quick-pickled veggies.

FOR THE PICKLED CARROTS AND RADISHES:

1 cup shredded carrots (about 2 medium carrots)

¼ cup sliced red onions

¼ cup shredded radishes

¼ cup white balsamic vinegar

FOR THE SPICED POTATOES:

4 Yukon Gold potatoes (about 1 pound), peeled, quartered lengthwise, and cut into 1-inch pieces

½ teaspoon kosher salt

1 tablespoon extra-virgin olive oil

⅓ cup diced yellow onions

1 clove garlic, minced

½ teaspoon grated fresh ginger

1 tablespoon tomato paste

½ teaspoon ground coriander

½ teaspoon ground cumin

½ teaspoon garam masala

½ teaspoon turmeric powder

Kosher salt and freshly ground black pepper

FOR ASSEMBLY:

4 (10-inch) flour tortillas

2 cups baby spinach leaves

¼ cup chopped fresh cilantro

Chutney of choice, for serving (optional)

Make the quick-pickled veggies:

1. Put the carrots, red onions, radishes, and vinegar in a glass bowl. Toss to evenly coat and let sit for about 20 minutes.

Meanwhile, make the spiced potatoes:

2. Place the potatoes in a large saucepan and add enough water to cover them by about 1 inch. Stir in the salt. Bring to a boil and cook the potatoes until fork-tender, about 5 minutes. Reserve ¼ cup of the cooking water, then drain the potatoes and set both aside.

3. Heat the olive oil in a large skillet over medium-low heat. Add the onions, garlic, and ginger and cook until the onions are translucent, about 5 minutes. Stir in the tomato paste, coriander, cumin, garam masala, and turmeric and cook for 30 seconds to release the fragrance of the spices.

4. Add the potatoes and reserved cooking water to the skillet and season to taste with salt and pepper. Cook until the water has evaporated and the potatoes are fully tender.

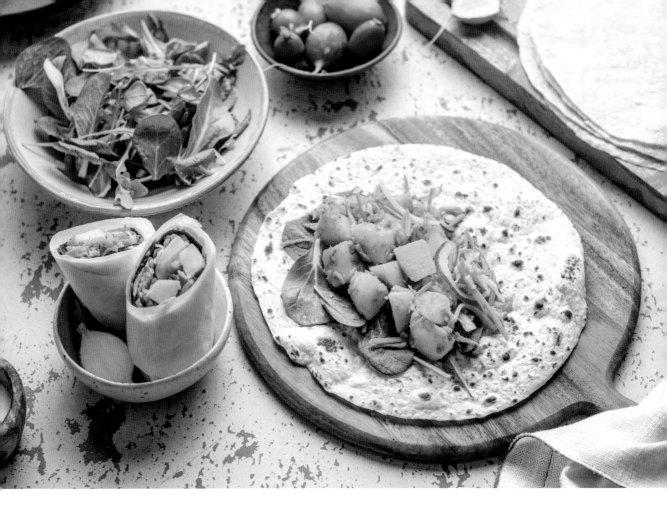

Assemble the wraps:

5. Heat each tortilla in a hot skillet for about 1 minute per side (or as directed on the package) to make it malleable. Arrange the spinach leaves in an even layer and top with the potatoes, pickled carrots and radishes, and a sprinkling of cilantro. Fold in the sides of each tortilla and roll them up burrito style.

6. Enjoy immediately, served with chutney, if you wish.

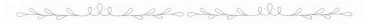

NOTE

For these wraps, I tend to go with tamarind or mango chutney, but feel free to use whatever chutney you like best or to experiment with different flavors.

Yield: 4 servings

Prep Time: 20 minutes, plus 1 hour to rest dough

Cook Time: 45 minutes

Roasted Vegetable Galette

Most people think of galettes for dessert, but I love a savory galette on occasion. Loaded with roasted vegetables, this galette can be an appetizer, served with a bowl of soup or a fresh salad, or a simple cozy meal on its own.

FOR THE DOUGH:

1 cup all-purpose flour, plus more for the work surface

½ teaspoon salt

½ cup (1 stick) unsalted butter, frozen

¼ cup ice water

FOR THE ROASTED VEGETABLES:

1½ cups diced butternut squash

1 cup broccoli florets

1 cup quartered cremini or white mushrooms

1 cup diced zucchini

1 cup diced yellow squash

½ cup diced red onions

½ cup chopped red bell peppers

2 cloves garlic, minced

2 tablespoons extra-virgin olive oil

1 teaspoon herbes de Provence

Kosher salt and freshly ground black pepper

FOR THE FILLING AND ASSEMBLY:

1 smoked chicken sausage link, quartered lengthwise and sliced

⅓ cup crumbled feta cheese

Extra-virgin olive oil

1 large egg

1 tablespoon water

Kosher salt and freshly ground black pepper

Grated Parmigiano-Reggiano cheese, for serving

Fresh thyme, for garnish (optional)

Make the dough:

1. In a medium bowl, stir together the flour and salt with a fork. Grate the butter with a box grater and add it to the flour mixture. Using your fingers, begin to work the butter into the flour until you have coarse crumbs.

2. Stir in the water 1 tablespoon at a time, using the fork to incorporate it and pinching the dough together with your fingers to check it; when the dough sticks together when pinched, it's sufficiently moistened. Take care not to make the dough too wet. You can also do this task with a food processor if you wish. Do not overwork the dough—you want to see bits of butter within it, and it will still be rather shaggy and loose.

3. Turn the dough out onto a lightly floured surface and use your hands to bring it together into a ball, but be careful not to overwork it. Wrap it in plastic wrap, form it into a disk, and refrigerate for at least an hour or overnight.

(recipe continues on page 89)

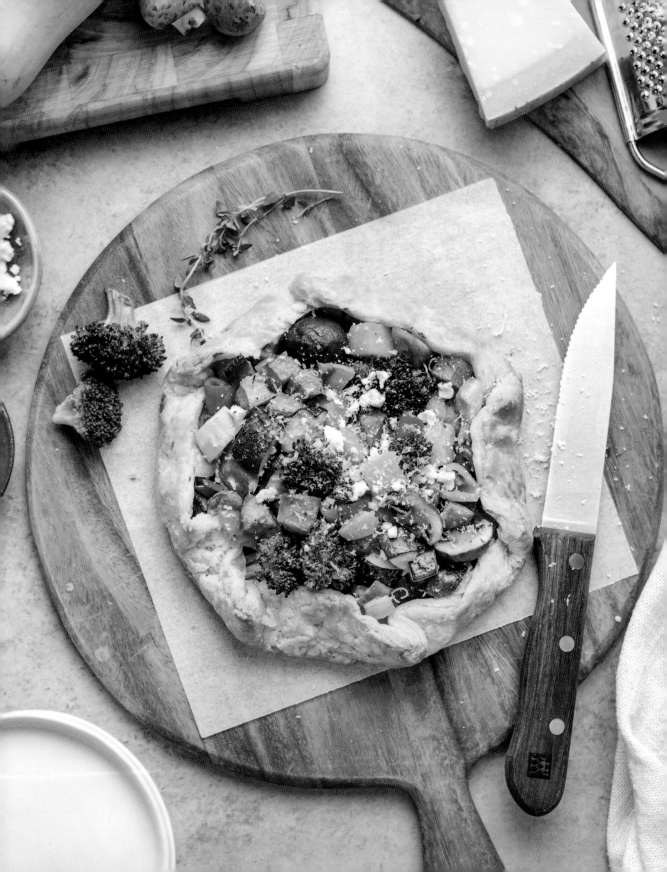

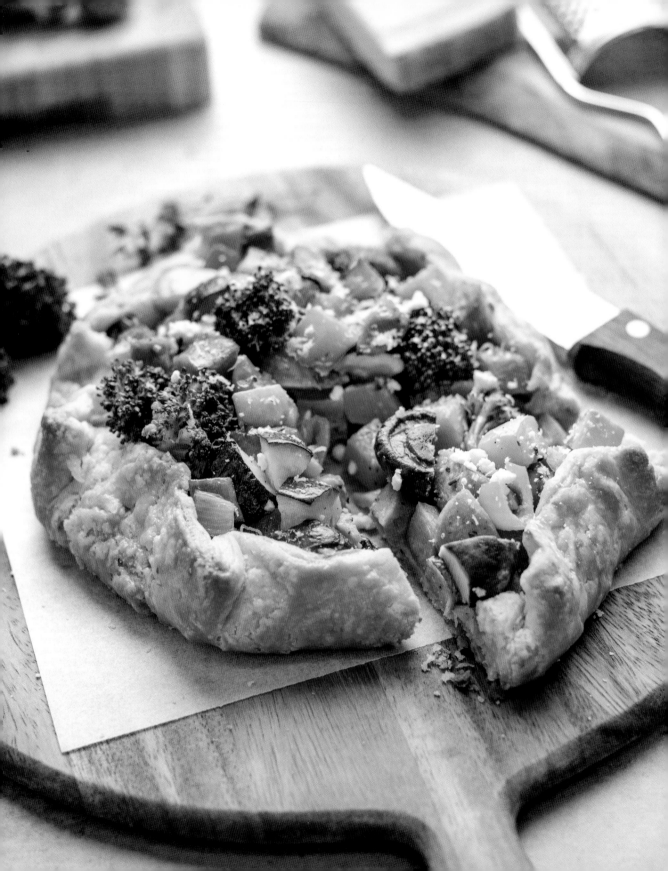

Roast the vegetables:

4. Preheat the oven to 425°F with a rack placed in the center of the oven. Line a sheet pan with parchment paper or aluminum foil.

5. Spread the vegetables on the prepared pan. Sprinkle the garlic on top, drizzle with the olive oil, and season with the herbes de Provence and a generous pinch each of salt and pepper. Use your hands to toss the vegetables, making sure they are evenly coated with the oil and seasonings.

6. Roast the vegetables for 15 minutes, or until they are just about fork-tender.

Make the galette:

7. Lower the oven temperature to 400°F.

8. On a sheet of parchment paper, roll the dough into a 12-inch disk about ¼ inch thick and place on a sheet pan.

9. Arrange the roasted vegetables and sausage on the dough, leaving a 2-inch perimeter. Sprinkle the feta cheese on top of the filling. Lightly drizzle the filling with a touch of olive oil and lightly season with salt and pepper.

10. Fold the edges of the dough up onto the filling, pleating it as you make your way around the galette. Refrigerate the galette for 10 minutes.

11. Whisk together the egg and water. Lightly brush the dough with the egg wash. Bake the galette for 25 to 30 minutes, or until the crust is golden brown.

12. Remove from the oven and sprinkle the galette with grated Parmigiano-Reggiano cheese. Let it cool slightly before slicing. Enjoy warm, garnished with thyme, if desired.

Yield: 4 servings

Prep Time: 15 minutes

Cook Time: 7 minutes

Gyro Flatbread *with* Cucumber Salad

One of the things I miss the most about the Greek diners of my New York childhood is the gyros! The intoxicating scent of roasted lamb twirling on its axis, and the way the knife would glide expertly, shaving ribbons into a veggie-packed pita—I was mesmerized by it all. This flatbread is my quick and easy way to satisfy that craving without hopping on a plane.

8 ounces ground lamb

¼ cup finely chopped yellow onions (about ½ medium onion)

1 clove garlic, minced

¾ teaspoon kosher salt

¾ teaspoon dried marjoram leaves

¼ teaspoon dried oregano leaves

¼ teaspoon dried rosemary leaves

⅛ teaspoon freshly ground black pepper

4 teaspoons extra-virgin olive oil, divided, plus more for brushing the breads

4 flatbreads, such as naan

1 cup sliced cucumbers

2 Campari tomatoes, chopped in 1-inch pieces (see Note)

½ cup sliced red onions

1 tablespoon fresh lemon juice

2 teaspoons white wine vinegar

½ cup tzatziki, homemade (page 76) or store-bought, plus more for serving

¼ cup crumbled feta cheese

½ cup mixed baby greens, for garnish (optional)

Fresh herbs (such as dill, mint, or parsley), for garnish

1. Preheat the oven to 400°F with a rack placed in the center of the oven.

2. Mix the lamb, onions, garlic, salt, marjoram, oregano, rosemary, and pepper in a bowl until well combined.

3. Heat 2 teaspoons of the olive oil in a medium skillet over medium heat. Add the lamb mixture and cook, breaking up the meat into bite-sized chunks, for about 7 minutes, until the meat is fully cooked and browned.

4. Meanwhile, lightly brush the flatbreads with olive oil, place on a sheet pan, and toast in the oven.

5. Toss the cucumbers, tomatoes, and red onions in a bowl with the remaining 2 teaspoons of olive oil, the lemon juice, and vinegar.

6. Spread the tzatziki on top of the toasted flatbreads and top with the lamb, cucumber salad, feta, baby greens (if using), and fresh herbs. Serve immediately with extra tzatziki.

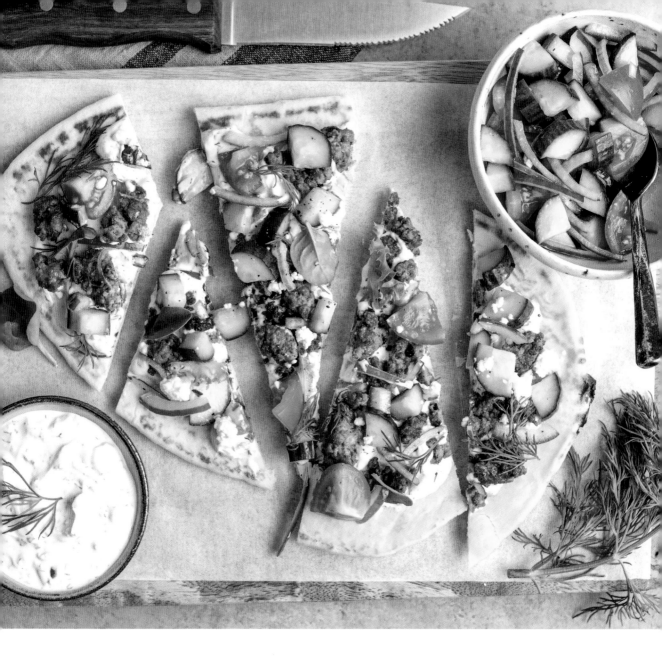

NOTE

Known as cocktail tomatoes, Campari tomatoes are small to medium-sized tomatoes (larger than cherry tomatoes but smaller than beefsteak tomatoes) that are prized for their sweet flavor. If you can't find Campari tomatoes, use your favorite variety—the sweeter and fresher, the better!

Avocado Toast *with* Eggs *and* Bacon

Yield: 4 servings

Prep Time: 5 minutes

Cook Time: 10 minutes

Is avocado toast passé? Never. At least not in California! It will always be a trend where avocados are plentiful. There's always a bowl of avocados on my kitchen counter, and I eat some form of avocado toast nearly every day! Add some eggs and bacon and you've got one of my favorite breakfasts that will fuel you up for the day.

4 slices hearty bread

2 ripe avocados, halved, pitted, and peeled

Kosher salt and freshly ground black pepper

2 slices bacon

2 teaspoons extra-virgin olive oil

4 large eggs

¼ cup crumbled feta cheese (optional)

1 cup microgreens

1. Toast the bread.

2. Mash the avocados in a bowl and spread on the toasted bread. Season with a pinch each of salt and pepper.

3. Cook the bacon in a large nonstick skillet over medium heat until crispy. Chop the bacon and sprinkle it over the avocado toast.

4. Wipe the skillet clean, then pour in the olive oil and set over low heat. Crack the eggs into the skillet, cover with a lid, and fry sunny-side-up for 2 minutes for runny yolks, or longer if you prefer more well-done yolks. Season with salt and pepper to taste.

5. Top the toast with the eggs, feta cheese (if using), and microgreens and enjoy!

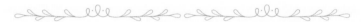

NOTE

There are various ways to toast the bread. The simplest, of course, is to toast it in a toaster. You can also do it under the oven broiler or in a hot skillet on the stovetop. For the oven or stovetop method, you can lightly brush the bread with a touch of olive oil or butter before toasting, but this is purely optional.

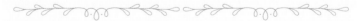

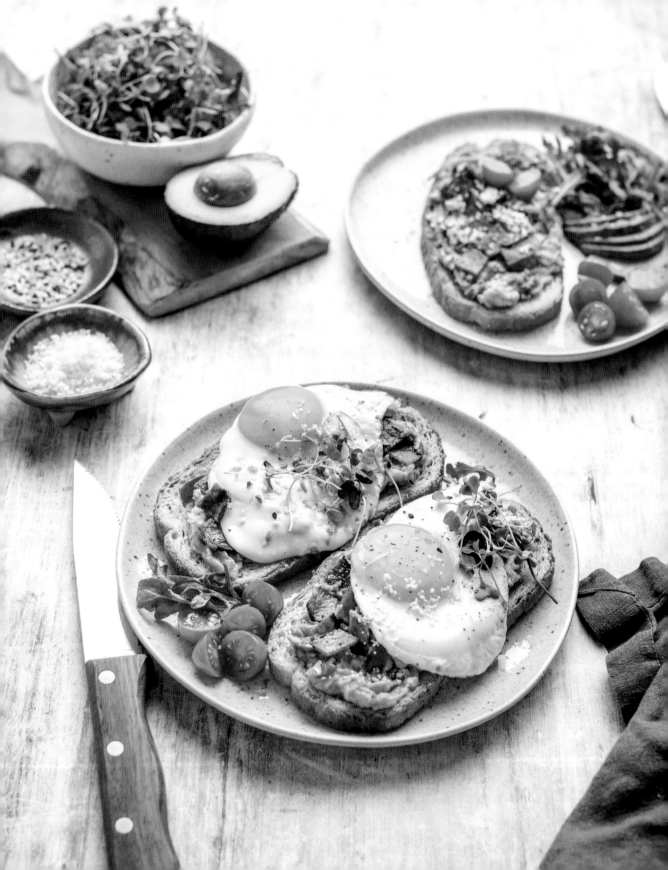

Roasted Winter Squash, Kale, *and* Turkey Bacon Pizza

Yield: 4 servings

Prep Time: 15 minutes

Cook Time: 30 minutes

Friday is pizza night at our house—there's nothing better than ending the week with doughy homemade goodness! Sometimes we fire up the pizza oven in the backyard, but if we need a quick fix, we make pizzas in the oven. Here, I give instructions for both methods. Either way, this is one of my favorite pizzas to make. If you've never tried adding butternut squash to pizza, I hope this recipe convinces you!

1½ cups ½-inch-diced butternut squash

3 cloves garlic, peel intact

1½ tablespoons extra-virgin olive oil, plus more for oiling the pan and brushing the dough

Kosher salt and freshly ground black pepper

1 cup destemmed and chopped kale

½ cup whole milk ricotta

½ cup fresh (soft) goat cheese or crumbled feta

1 (16-ounce) prepared pizza dough ball

¼ cup pesto

¼ cup thinly sliced red onions, divided

2 slices turkey bacon, cut into ½-inch pieces

1. Preheat the oven to 400°F. Lightly grease a baking sheet with olive oil.

2. Place the butternut squash and garlic cloves on a sheet pan, drizzle with the olive oil, season generously with salt and pepper, and toss well, using your hands to evenly coat the squash. Roast for 10 to 12 minutes, or until the squash is just about fork-tender.

3. Remove the squash from the oven and push it to one side of the sheet pan. Drop the kale on the other side of the pan and toss to coat the greens with the residual olive oil. Set aside.

4. Squeeze the roasted garlic out of the peel into a small bowl and mash with a fork. Mix in the ricotta and goat cheese and season with ½ teaspoon each of salt and pepper.

5. Raise the oven temperature to 475°F with a rack placed in the lower half of the oven.

6. On a floured surface, roll out the pizza dough until it's about ¼ inch thick and, if making a round pizza, 12 inches in diameter (or roll it to your desired shape). Transfer to the prepared baking sheet. Using your fingertips, lightly press some dimples into the dough, then fold the edge of the dough over all around the perimeter to create a ridge (this will prevent the cheeses from oozing out). Brush the edge of the dough lightly with olive oil.

7. Spread the pesto onto the dough, leaving a 1-inch margin around the perimeter. Spread the ricotta mixture over the dough and top with half of the red onions, all of the squash, and half of the kale. Scatter the bacon on top.

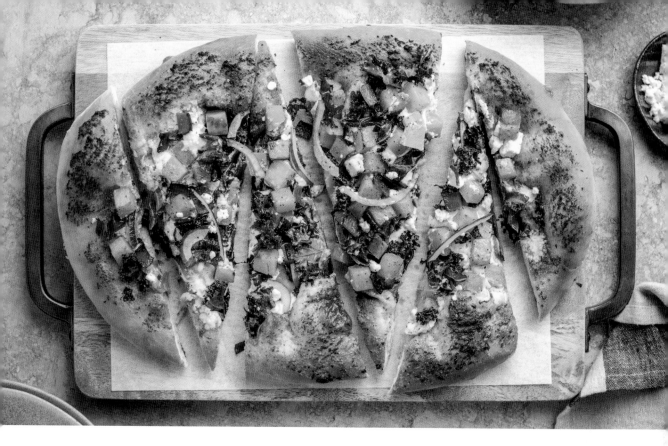

8. Bake the pizza for 13 to 14 minutes, then top with the remaining kale and bake until the crust is golden, another 2 to 3 minutes.

9. Top the pizza with the remaining onions, slice, and serve.

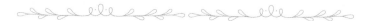

NOTES

Once in a while, I love to use our wood-fired pizza oven—nothing compares to the crisp charred crust, and pizzas take mere seconds to cook! If you have a pizza oven, here's how to make this recipe:

Preheat the pizza oven following the manufacturer's instructions.

Complete Steps 1 through 7 as written, forming the pizza on a pizza paddle dusted with cornmeal. Slide the pizza into the pizza oven and bake for 30 to 40 seconds, then top with the remaining kale and rotate. Bake for an additional 30 to 40 seconds, until the crust is evenly cooked. Complete Step 9.

Roasted Eggplant Flatbread

Yield: 2 servings

Prep Time: 5 minutes

Cook Time: 15 minutes

Store-bought naan is a staple in my kitchen, and it's my shortcut to quick and easy flatbreads. This one is an old favorite, made with roasted eggplant, juicy tomatoes, and pesto—basically, summer on a flatbread!

1 small eggplant

¼ cup extra-virgin olive oil

Kosher salt and freshly ground black pepper

1 naan (see Note)

1 cup pesto

1 large or 2 medium tomatoes, sliced into ¼-inch rounds

1 cup crumbled feta cheese

2 tablespoons chopped fresh flat-leaf parsley

1. Preheat the oven to 400°F with a rack placed in the center of the oven. Line two sheet pans with parchment paper.

2. Slice the eggplant crosswise into ¼-inch rounds; you should have about 6 rounds. Lay the rounds on one of the prepared pans.

3. Brush the eggplant on both sides with the olive oil, lightly season on both sides with salt and pepper, and roast for about 10 minutes, until the eggplant is just fork-tender. Remove from the oven but leave the oven on.

4. Place the naan on the other prepared sheet pan. Spread a layer of pesto on the naan. Arrange the eggplant and tomato rounds on the naan in a single layer, slightly overlapping. Lightly season with a pinch each of salt and pepper, sprinkle with the feta cheese, and pop the pan in the oven for 4 to 5 minutes, or until the tomatoes have wilted, the cheese has softened, and the naan is toasted.

5. Remove the flatbread from the oven, sprinkle with the parsley, and enjoy immediately.

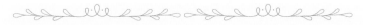

NOTE

These days, it is much easier to find naan at your local grocer—look for it in the bread or freezer aisles. If you can't find naan, feel free to substitute two pita breads.

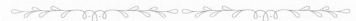

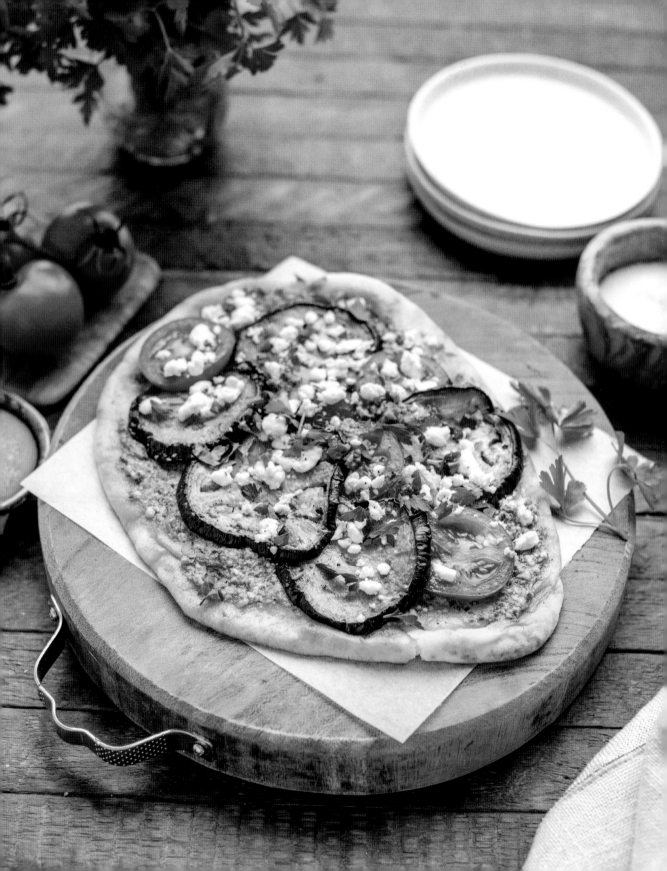

Mini Eggplant Pizzas

Yield: 4 servings

Prep Time: 5 minutes

Cook Time: 18 minutes

I was at the doctor's office when I first found out about eggplant pizzas—turns out my nurse is an excellent cook and nutritionist! I immediately started experimenting and found I love making them with sun-dried tomato pesto for an extra flavor punch. These little pizzas are individually sized and perfect as an appetizer.

1 medium eggplant, sliced in ½-inch rounds

2 tablespoons extra-virgin olive oil

Kosher salt and freshly ground black pepper

1 cup sun-dried tomato pesto

2 ounces Halloumi cheese, sliced

6 ounces mozzarella cheese, sliced

¼ cup pitted Castelvetrano olives, halved

¼ cup cherry or grape tomatoes, halved

Fresh basil sprigs, for garnish

1. Preheat the oven to 450°F with a rack placed in the center of the oven. Line a sheet pan with parchment paper.

2. Brush the eggplant rounds on both sides with the olive oil and lightly season on both sides with salt and pepper. Roast for about 10 minutes, until the eggplant is just fork-tender.

3. Flip the eggplant rounds over and spread a layer of sun-dried tomato pesto on each one. Top the rounds with the Halloumi and mozzarella cheeses and some olives and tomatoes.

4. Bake the eggplant pizzas for another 8 minutes, or until the cheeses have melted.

5. Garnish the eggplant pizzas with fresh basil and serve immediately.

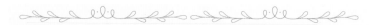

NOTE

Castelvetrano olives are one of my favorites. Delicious straight out of the jar, they are known for their mild, sweet flavor and buttery smooth texture. If you can't find Castelvetrano olives, substitute Manzanillas, black olives, or whatever variety you like best.

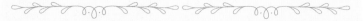

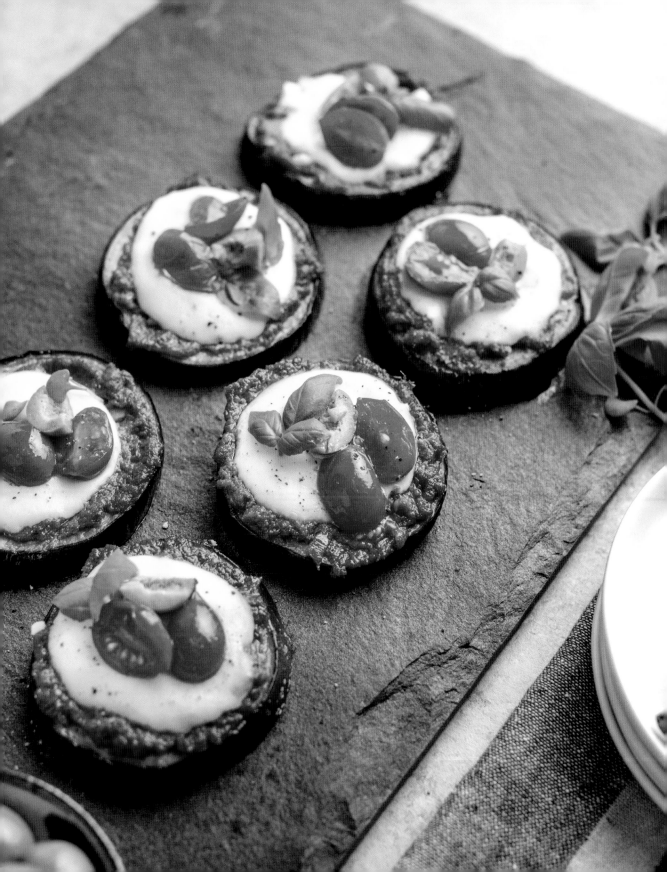

Veggie Bacon Burgers

Yield: 6 servings

Prep Time: 15 minutes

Cook Time: 20 minutes

My daughter and I are constantly trying new veggie burger recipes—whether it's at a restaurant or at home. She's a tough critic, so getting her thumbs-up can be pretty challenging. Luckily, these veggie burgers have her approval!

1 (15-ounce) can black beans, drained and rinsed

½ cup mashed, cooked sweet potato (see Note)

2 tablespoons plus 2 teaspoons extra-virgin olive oil, divided

⅓ cup diced yellow onions

2 cloves garlic, minced

¼ teaspoon ground cumin

¼ teaspoon paprika

⅛ teaspoon chili powder

½ cup Italian breadcrumbs

¼ cup shredded Halloumi cheese

1 large egg

2 teaspoons Worcestershire sauce

1 teaspoon soy sauce

6 hamburger buns, for serving

6 slices bacon, cooked, for serving

SUGGESTED TOPPINGS:

Mayonnaise and/or other condiments of choice

Lettuce leaves

Cheese slices

Sliced red onion

Pickles

Tomato slices

1. In a medium bowl, mash the beans and sweet potato together with a fork or potato masher. The ingredients should be well combined, but the beans should still have some texture.

2. Heat 2 teaspoons of the olive oil in a large skillet over medium-low heat. Add the onions and garlic and cook until the onions are translucent, about 5 minutes. Add the mixture to the bowl of mashed beans and sweet potato and set the skillet aside.

3. To the bean mixture, add the cumin, paprika, chili powder, breadcrumbs, Halloumi cheese, egg, Worcestershire sauce, and soy sauce. Mix with a fork until well combined.

4. Using a ½-cup measuring cup, portion and form the mixture into six patties about 3½ inches in diameter (or refer to the size of your hamburger buns and size the patties appropriately). It helps to use lightly dampened hands to form the patties.

5. Heat 1 tablespoon of the olive oil in the same skillet over medium heat. When the oil is hot, add half of the burger patties to the pan, making sure there is ample space between them. Cook the burgers for 3 to 4 minutes per side, until they are golden and crispy on the outside and heated through. Repeat with the remaining tablespoon of olive oil and burger patties.

6. Serve the burgers on the hamburger buns topped with the bacon and your desired condiments and toppings.

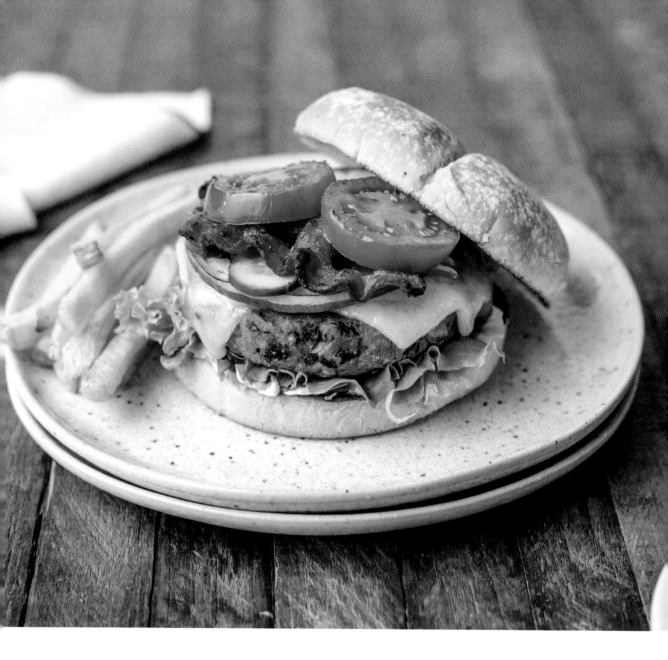

NOTE

When preparing mashed, cooked sweet potato for recipes like this one, I like to cook the sweet potato in the microwave; you can find instructions for doing so on page 54. For the ½ cup of mashed sweet potato used in this recipe, you will need 1 small sweet potato.

Yield: 8 to 10 servings

Prep Time: 10 minutes

Cook Time: 6 or 10 hours, depending on heat level used

Lentil Pulled Pork Sandwiches

The scent of the pork braising in a slow cooker is guaranteed to get you tiptoeing into the kitchen looking to sneak a bite, but try to resist until you mix in the hearty lentils—you'll get a lightened-up version that still has the meaty pulled pork flavor you love!

2 medium yellow onions, thinly sliced

4 cloves garlic, smashed with the side of a knife

1 tablespoon chili powder

1 tablespoon kosher salt

1 teaspoon ground coriander

1 teaspoon ground cumin

1 teaspoon brown sugar

1 (3-pound) boneless pork shoulder/butt

12 ounces lime soda

6 ounces ginger beer

1 cup chicken stock

2 cups barbecue sauce, plus more for serving

Sriracha sauce

Freshly ground black pepper

FOR THE LENTILS:

1 cup green lentils, rinsed and drained

2½ cups water

½ teaspoon kosher salt

1 tablespoon extra-virgin olive oil

½ cup diced yellow onions (about ½ medium onion)

Reserved spice rub (from above)

Burger buns, toasted, for serving

Shredded red cabbage, for serving

Shredded carrots, for serving

1. Place the sliced onions and garlic in a 5-quart or larger slow cooker.

2. In a small bowl, combine the chili powder, salt, coriander, cumin, and brown sugar. Set aside 3 tablespoons of the spice rub for the lentils.

3. Rub the pork shoulder on all sides with the rest of the spice rub. Place the seasoned pork shoulder, fat side up, on the bed of onions and garlic in the slow cooker.

4. Pour in the lime soda, ginger beer, and chicken stock. Cover and cook for 6 hours on high or 10 hours on low, until the meat is fork-tender and coming apart. If you can, rotate the pork shoulder once during cooking.

5. When the pork has about a half hour left to cook, place the lentils, water, and salt in a small saucepan. Bring to a boil over medium-high heat, then reduce the heat to low and simmer for 25 minutes, or until the lentils are tender. Drain the lentils.

6. Heat the olive oil in a large skillet over medium-low heat. Add the diced onions and cook until translucent, about 5 minutes. Stir in the drained lentils and reserved spice rub. Cook for another 5 minutes, then set aside.

7. Carefully transfer the cooked pork to a cutting board. Shred the meat using two forks; discard any fat. Place the pulled pork in a bowl with the cooked lentils and stir in the barbecue sauce. Season to taste with Sriracha (for heat), salt, and pepper.

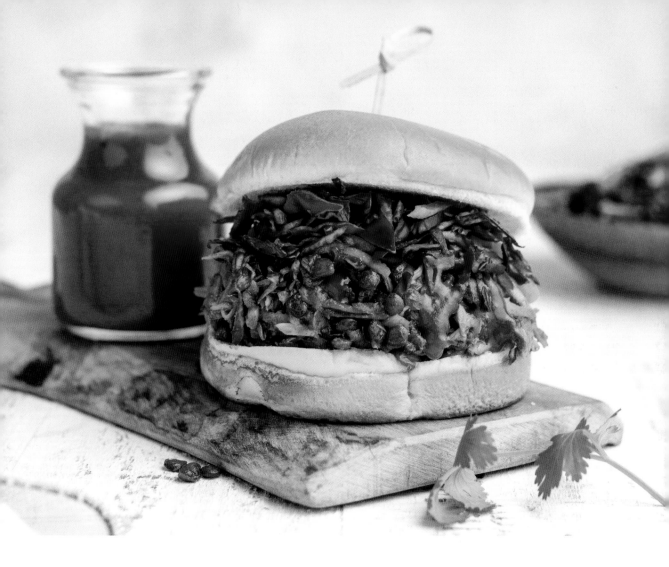

8. Serve the lentil pulled pork on toasted buns with additional barbecue sauce, shredded cabbage, and shredded carrots.

NOTE

Many pulled pork recipes call for a dark soda, which adds caramelization and sweetness to the pork. I've also been known to use beer in my pulled pork, which tenderizes the meat. In this version, I use both ginger beer and lime soda, which adds a similar caramelization, just a light touch of sweetness, and a ginger-citrus undertone.

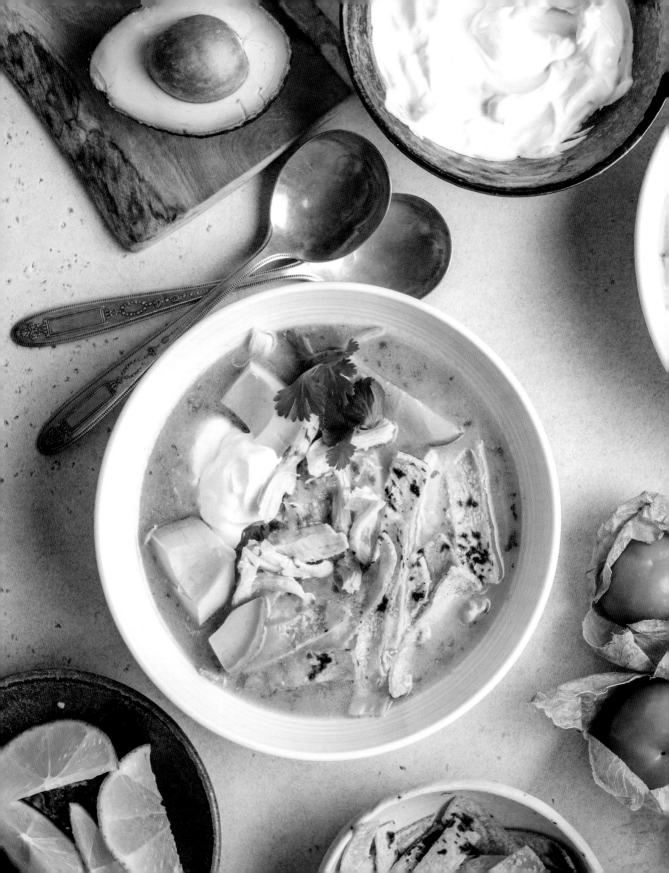

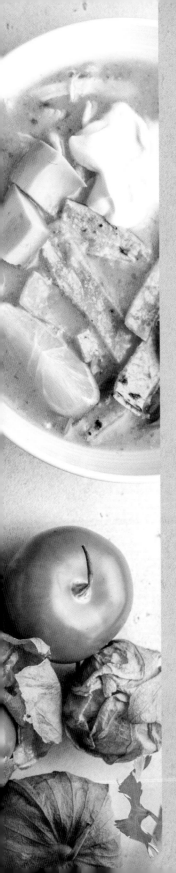

Soups

Italian Wedding Soup

Yield: 8 servings

Prep Time: 20 minutes

Cook Time: 30 minutes

I love sneaking in extra veggies anywhere I can, and meatballs, to me, are the ideal vehicle to subtly deliver more greens without anyone suspecting. A little extra helping of kale is packed into the flavorful meatballs in this classic dish, guaranteeing that we eat more veggies without even really trying.

FOR THE MEATBALLS:

1 small yellow onion, grated

⅓ cup minced kale

1 large egg

1 teaspoon minced garlic

1 teaspoon dried parsley

1 teaspoon kosher salt

¼ teaspoon freshly ground black pepper

⅓ cup panko breadcrumbs

½ cup grated Parmigiano-Reggiano cheese, plus more for serving

8 ounces 85% lean ground beef

8 ounces ground pork

FOR THE SOUP:

2 tablespoons extra-virgin olive oil

1 cup minced yellow onions (about 1 medium onion)

1 cup ¼-inch-diced carrots (about 3 medium carrots)

1 cup ¼-inch diced celery (2 to 3 medium stalks)

10 cups chicken stock (see Notes)

1 cup small pasta, such as orzo, acini di pepe, or tubetini

Kosher salt and freshly ground black pepper

8 ounces kale, chopped (see Notes)

Make the meatballs:

1. In a medium bowl, stir together the onion, minced kale, egg, garlic, parsley, salt, pepper, and breadcrumbs. Add the cheese and ground meats and combine using your hands or a fork. Using about a heaping teaspoon portion, roll the mixture into meatballs; this will yield about 40 meatballs. Set aside on a sheet pan. This step can be done in advance (see Notes).

Make the soup:

2. Heat the olive oil in a Dutch oven or soup pot over medium heat. Add the onions, carrots, and celery and sauté until the onions are translucent, about 7 minutes.

3. Pour in the chicken stock and bring to a boil. Add the pasta and meatballs, return to a boil, and cook until the pasta is al dente and the meatballs are cooked through, about 10 minutes.

4. Taste the broth and adjust the seasoning to your liking with salt and pepper. Stir in the chopped kale and simmer for a couple of minutes more, until the kale is just wilted but still a vibrant green.

5. Ladle into bowls and serve with a little extra grated cheese.

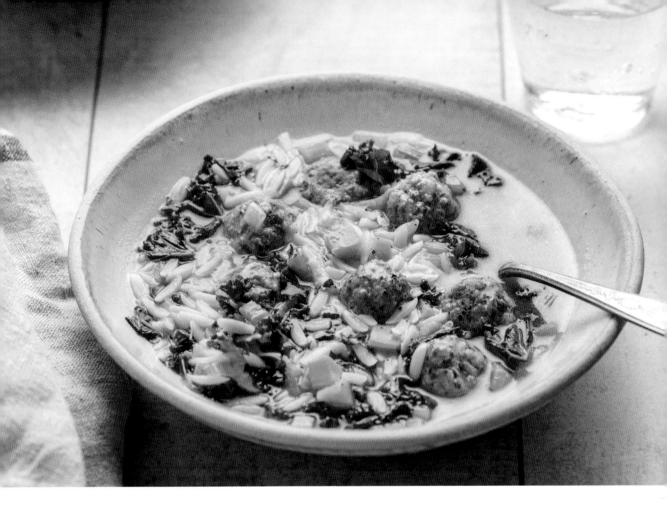

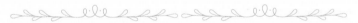

NOTES

The meatballs can be made a day in advance. Form them and store on a sheet pan covered with plastic wrap in the refrigerator. For longer-term storage, arrange the meatballs on a sheet pan so they are not touching and freeze until solid. Transfer to an airtight container such as a freezer bag and freeze for up to 2 months.

Given the large quantity of stock used here, this is the perfect recipe to use homemade if you have some on hand; not only does homemade stock taste better, but it's generally more nutritious. If you don't, store-bought chicken stock is just fine.

The greens in this recipe are flexible. A traditional Italian wedding soup often uses escarole, and most recipes call for spinach. I prefer using kale for its heartiness and nutrients, but feel free to use the greens you have available to you.

Creamy Cauliflower Soup *with* Pancetta

Yield: 5 servings
Prep Time: 8 minutes
Cook Time: 30 minutes

There's nothing cozier than a creamy soup. What I love about this one is that most of the creaminess comes from the cauliflower itself. This is a soup that won't weigh you down, even with the addition of milk (the secret ingredient to provide silkiness). Crispy pancetta is the perfect garnish!

2 teaspoons extra-virgin olive oil, plus more for garnish

2 ounces diced pancetta

1 cup finely chopped yellow onions (about 1 medium onion)

Kosher salt

1 small head cauliflower, cut into florets

3 cups chicken stock

2 cups whole milk

Freshly ground black pepper

2 tablespoons chopped fresh flat-leaf parsley, for garnish (optional)

1. Heat the olive oil in a Dutch oven or soup pot over medium heat. Add the pancetta and cook for 4 minutes, or until crispy. Remove with a slotted spoon to a paper towel–lined plate.

2. Add the onions to the pot, season with a pinch of salt, and cook until wilted and translucent, 5 to 7 minutes.

3. Add the cauliflower florets and chicken stock. Increase the heat to medium-high, bring to a boil, and then lower the heat to a simmer. Cover and let the soup bubble for 10 minutes, or until the cauliflower is fork-tender. Stir in the milk.

4. Purée the soup in a blender, working in batches if necessary. If you have one, an immersion blender makes this task easier.

5. Return the soup to the pot and season to taste with salt and pepper. Reheat the soup over low heat for 3 to 5 minutes, or until nice and hot.

6. Serve hot, garnished with the pancetta and a sprinkle of parsley, if desired.

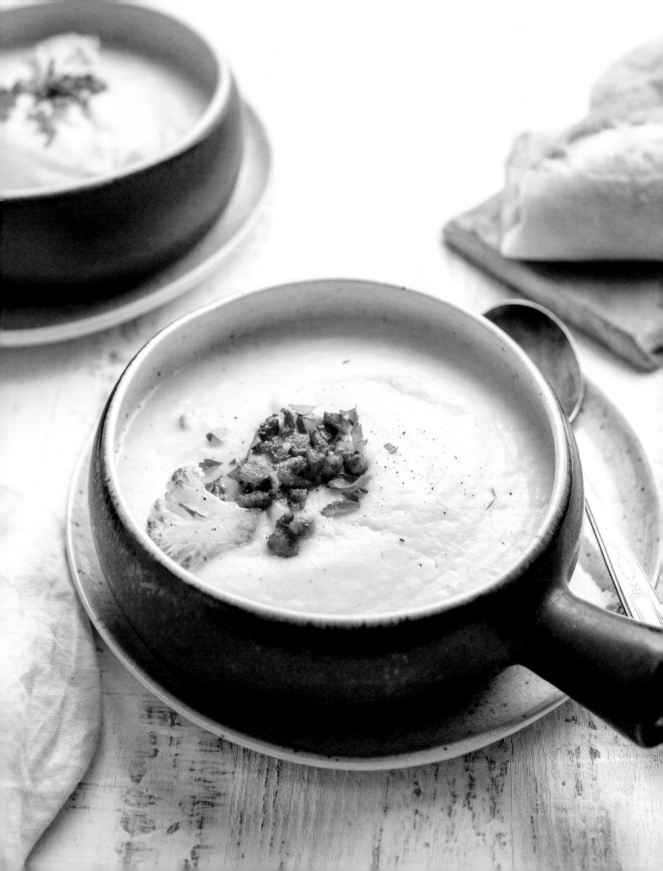

Thai Curry Butternut Squash Lentil Soup

Yield: 6 servings

Prep Time: 10 minutes

Cook Time: 40 minutes

When I need something warm and comforting, this soup checks all the boxes. Lentil soup is one of the coziest soups around, and when made with butternut squash, it has a lovely creaminess without the cream. A touch of Thai curry adds an extra layer of warmth to this soup.

2 tablespoons extra-virgin olive oil

1 cup finely chopped yellow onions (about 1 medium onion)

1 teaspoon minced garlic

1 teaspoon grated fresh ginger

1 tablespoon red curry paste

4 cups roughly chopped butternut squash

1 cup red lentils

1 teaspoon kosher salt

6 cups vegetable stock

½ cup canned light coconut milk

1 teaspoon Sriracha sauce, plus more for garnish if desired

Freshly ground black pepper

Fresh cilantro, for garnish

1. Heat the olive oil in a Dutch oven or soup pot over medium-low heat. Add the onions, garlic, and ginger and cook until the onions have wilted, about 3 minutes. Stir in the curry paste and cook for another minute to toast the spices.

2. Add the butternut squash, lentils, salt, and vegetable stock and bring to a boil. Lower the heat to a simmer, then cover the pot and cook, stirring periodically, for about 30 minutes, until the squash and lentils are tender.

3. Using an immersion blender, blend the soup until the squash is mostly or fully mashed, depending on your desired consistency—I like to keep it a little chunky. This can also be done by blending a portion of the soup in a blender and returning it to the pot.

4. Stir in the coconut milk and Sriracha and adjust the seasoning with salt and pepper to taste if necessary.

5. Garnish with cilantro and a drizzle of Sriracha (if you like heat). Serve immediately.

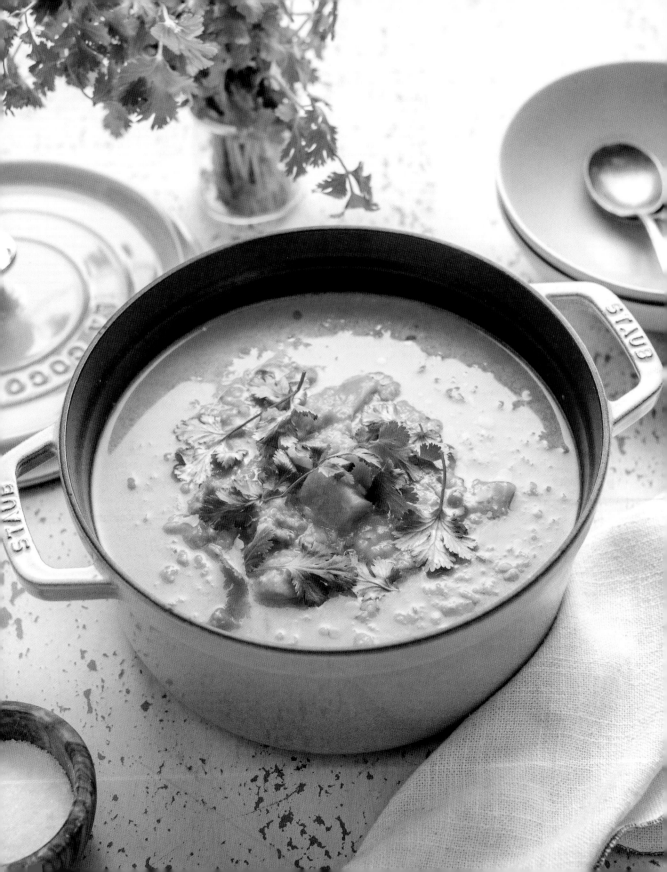

Veggie Miso Ramen

Yield: 2 servings
Prep Time: 25 minutes
Cook Time: 35 minutes

It doesn't matter the weather or the time of year—I can always go for a piping-hot bowl of ramen! When we traveled to Japan, I had an incredible vegetable ramen that I knew I had to recreate when I returned home. My version comes close, with a comforting broth, slurp-ready noodles, and as many veggies as my bowl can hold.

2 teaspoons untoasted sesame oil (unrefined)

½ cup minced shallots (about 1 large shallot)

1½ teaspoons minced garlic (about 2 cloves)

1 teaspoon grated fresh ginger

2 cups sliced mushrooms, such as shiitake or cremini

1 teaspoon soy sauce

2 teaspoons spicy chili paste, such as gochujang, or spicy bean paste, such as la doubanjiang (see Notes)

3 tablespoons white miso paste

4 cups chicken stock

Kosher salt and freshly ground black pepper

10 ounces ramen noodles

1 cup chopped curly kale

1 cup diced pan-fried firm tofu

½ cup canned corn kernels

½ cup shelled edamame

½ cup shredded carrots

¼ cup canned bamboo shoots

1 baby bok choy, quartered lengthwise

FOR GARNISH:

Sliced green onions

Furikake (see Notes)

Sesame seeds

2 soft-boiled eggs, sliced in half (optional)

1. Heat the sesame oil in a large saucepan over medium-low heat. Add the shallots, garlic, and ginger and cook until the shallots have wilted, about 3 minutes.

2. Add the mushrooms to the pan and increase the heat to medium-high. Stir in the soy sauce and cook until the mushrooms are tender, about 5 minutes.

3. Stir in the chili paste and miso paste, mixing them into the mushrooms.

4. Pour in the chicken stock and bring to a boil. Season to taste with salt and pepper. Lower the heat, cover, and let the soup simmer while you prepare the noodles.

5. Bring a large pot of water to a boil over high heat. Cook the ramen noodles according to the package directions. Drain and divide the noodles between two bowls.

6. Top the noodles with the kale, tofu, corn, edamame, carrots, bamboo shoots, and bok choy, then divide the hot broth between the bowls.

7. Garnish each bowl with some green onions, furikake, and sesame seeds and a soft-boiled egg, if using.

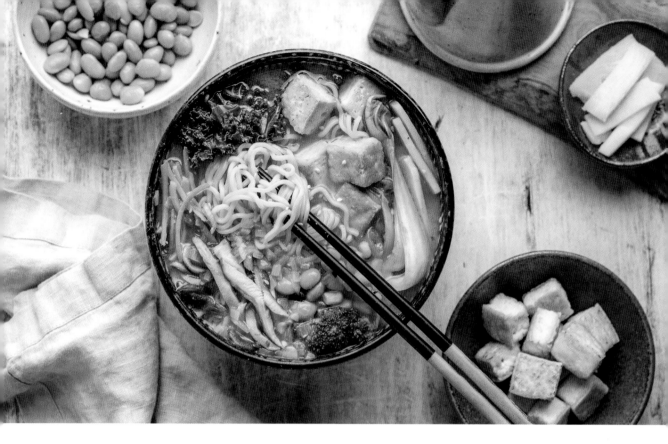

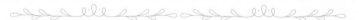

NOTES

The broth can be made ahead of time. Once fully cooled, store in an airtight container in the refrigerator for up to 3 days. Be sure to stir it well when you reheat it, as the miso may separate from the broth.

La doubanjiang is a spicy Chinese condiment made with fermented chili bean paste and red chili peppers that is popular in Sichuan cooking. You can find it at your local Asian market. Compared to gochujang, la doubanjiang has a punchier flavor, so take this into consideration when you season the ramen. (*Note:* At the market, you may find both doubanjiang and la doubanjiang—the la doubanjiang is the spicier of the two.)

Furikake is a Japanese condiment made with nori (seaweed), toasted sesame seeds, salt, sugar, and sometimes dried fish. Often sprinkled on dishes or cooked rice, it adds a delicious umami taste when sprinkled on ramen. You can find furikake at most Asian markets, and sometimes in the Asian section of the grocery store. If you have a Trader Joe's near you, they sell a wonderful furikake.

Yield: 4 servings
Prep Time: 10 minutes
Cook Time: 1 hour

Roasted Tomato Soup au Pistou

It wasn't until I was an adult that I appreciated the beauty of a good tomato soup—I think it was growing up believing that tomato soup came out of a can that kept me from trying it...that, and a strange idea that tomato soup must taste like warm ketchup! But once I learned how to coax the deep flavors from roasted, homegrown summer tomatoes, my life and outlook on tomato soup were forever changed. This soup, my son's favorite, is so simple to make. I love drizzling a pistou on top before serving—feel free to substitute pesto if you prefer! Either way, it's summer in a bowl.

FOR THE SOUP:

3 pounds tomatoes

6 cloves garlic, peel intact

2 medium shallots, halved

2 sprigs fresh thyme

2 tablespoons extra-virgin olive oil, plus more for garnish

Kosher salt and freshly ground black pepper

4 cups chicken stock or vegetable stock

1 bay leaf

1 teaspoon herbes de Provence

FOR THE PISTOU:

4 cloves garlic, roughly chopped

Kosher salt

2 cups fresh basil leaves

½ cup extra-virgin olive oil

Crusty bread, for serving

1. Preheat the oven to 400°F with a rack placed in the center of the oven.

2. Slice the tomatoes in half and arrange on a sheet pan with the garlic cloves, shallots, and thyme. Drizzle with the olive oil, give everything a toss to coat, and season liberally with salt and pepper. Roast until the tomatoes are soft and fragrant, the shallots are translucent, and the garlic is bursting from the peel, 20 to 25 minutes. This step can be done in advance if you like.

3. Remove and discard the garlic peels. Transfer the roasted tomatoes, garlic, shallots, and thyme to a Dutch oven or soup pot, along with all the juices.

4. Add the chicken stock, bay leaf, and herbes de Provence. Bring to a boil, then lower the heat and simmer uncovered for 30 minutes.

5. Remove the thyme stems and bay leaf. Use an immersion blender, or transfer to a blender (in batches), to pulse the soup until smooth. If you prefer a smoother soup, pass it through a sieve. Adjust the seasoning with salt and pepper and return the pot to low heat to keep the soup warm while you make the pistou.

6. Make the pistou: Using a mortar and pestle or a small food processor, mash the garlic and a pinch of salt to form a paste. Add the basil and mash/process until combined. Slowly add the olive oil in a stream, mixing to combine. Adjust the seasoning with salt to taste.

7. Serve the soup with a dollop of pistou, a drizzle of olive oil, and hot, crusty bread.

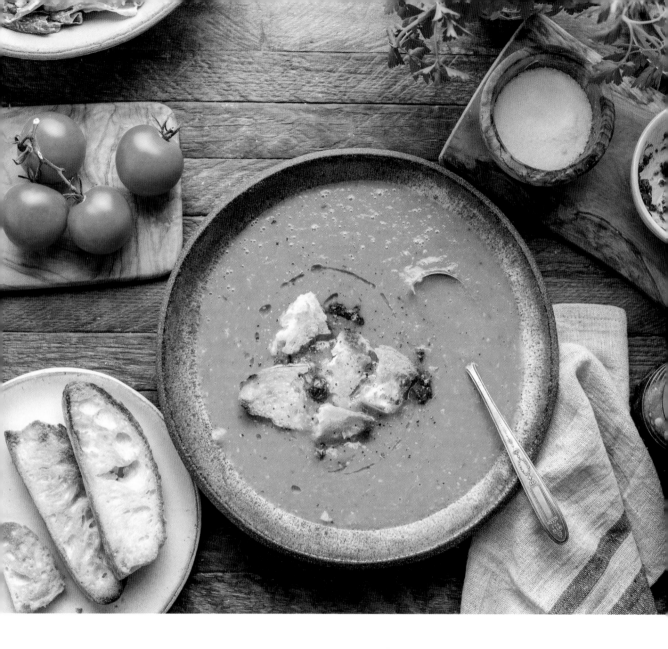

NOTE

Pistou is the French version of Italian pesto, but without the pine nuts. Some pistous use cheese and others do not, so I leave it up to you to decide. This simple sauce is made with garlic, salt, basil, and olive oil and adds a beautiful pop of flavor and a taste of the south of France to soups such as this and so much more.

Chicken Corn Soup

Yield: 4 servings

Prep Time: 10 minutes

Cook Time: 35 minutes

There's nothing more comforting than chicken soup, and I love this simple version with its pop of sweet corn kernels. It's like a chowder without the heaviness from cream. This recipe can be made with convenient frozen corn kernels or fresh corn; both options create a delicious soup. If you're using fresh corn, don't throw out the cobs—add them to the soup for extra corn flavor.

1 tablespoon extra-virgin olive oil

2 cups ½-inch diced carrots (about 4 medium carrots)

1 cup sliced celery (about 2 medium stalks)

2 quarts chicken stock

1 bone-in, skin-on split chicken breast (about 1 pound)

½ yellow onion, rinsed (leave the skin on)

2 cups fresh corn kernels (from 2 to 3 ears) or frozen corn kernels (reserve the cobs if using fresh)

Kosher salt and freshly ground black pepper

1. Heat the olive oil in a Dutch oven or soup pot over medium heat. Add the carrots and celery and cook until slightly softened, about 2 minutes.

2. Pour in the chicken stock and add the chicken breast, onion half, and trimmed corncobs if using fresh corn. Bring to a boil, then lower the heat to a gentle simmer, cover, and poach the chicken until cooked through, about 20 minutes.

3. When the chicken is cooked, take it out of the pot and let it cool slightly. When it is cool enough to handle, remove and discard the bone and skin. Shred the meat and return it to the soup. Remove and discard the onion and corn cobs, if used.

4. Stir the corn kernels into the soup and continue simmering until the corn is cooked and tender, about 5 minutes. Season to taste with salt and pepper. Serve immediately.

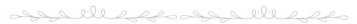

NOTES

When corn is in season, this is a wonderful way to enjoy the sweet, fresh kernels and get extra flavor from the cobs. If you find yourself with extra trimmed cobs, be sure to freeze them to add to soups like this one. I also love to keep frozen corn kernels on hand so I can make this cozy soup any time of year!

This soup is a wonderful base for other add-ins to make it heartier. Diced potatoes, orzo, rice, and noodles are great options for a more filling soup and can be added after the chicken is shredded and returned to the soup. Just be sure to add time to cook the add-ins as necessary. Adding uncooked rice or pasta to the soup will also require more liquid; add another 1 to 2 cups of broth to the soup.

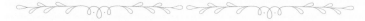

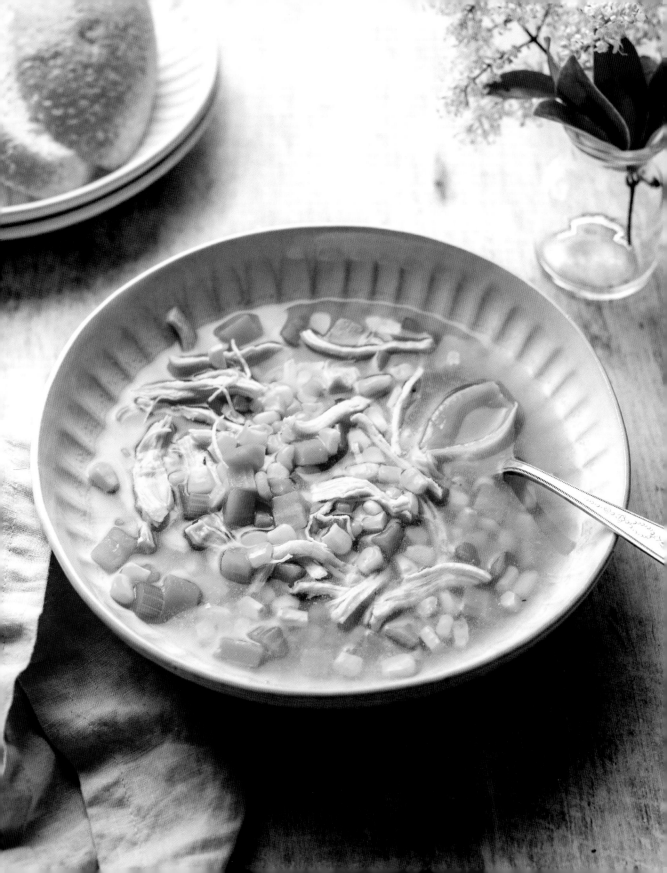

Thai-Style Chicken Noodle Vegetable Soup

Yield: 4 servings
Prep Time: 20 minutes
Cook Time: 30 minutes

I call this the green smoothie of chicken soups. Infused with the flavor of Thai green curry, it packs a nutritious punch from the kale that is blended into the broth, giving it an extra-vibrant shade of green. Top it with more veggies for a nourishing bowl!

8.8 ounces thin rice noodles

2 teaspoons extra-virgin olive oil

½ cup minced shallots (about 1 large shallot)

2 teaspoons minced garlic (2 to 3 cloves)

1 teaspoon grated fresh ginger

2 teaspoons green curry paste

3 cups chicken stock

8 ounces boneless, skinless chicken breast

1 cup canned light coconut milk

3 cups chopped kale, divided

½ teaspoon kosher salt

½ cup chopped fresh cilantro

Juice of ½ lime

Fish sauce or additional kosher salt

Freshly ground black pepper

4 lime wedges, for serving

TOPPINGS:

2 baby bok choy, halved and blanched

1 cup snow peas or sugar snap peas, blanched

1 cup bean sprouts

⅓ cup fresh cilantro leaves

⅓ cup fresh basil leaves, preferably Thai

¼ cup sliced green onions

1 jalapeño pepper, sliced

1. Prepare the noodles: Bring a large pot of water to a rolling boil. Season the water with salt, stir in the noodles, and turn off the heat. Let stand for 3 to 5 minutes, then drain the noodles and set aside.

2. Heat the olive oil in a medium saucepan over medium-low heat. Add the shallots and cook until translucent, 3 to 5 minutes. Stir in the garlic, ginger, and curry paste and cook for 30 seconds.

3. Add the chicken stock and chicken breast, increase the heat to medium, and slowly bring to a simmer. Cover the pan and simmer for 10 to 15 minutes, or until the chicken is cooked through.

4. Transfer the chicken to a plate and use two forks to shred the meat. Set aside.

5. Pour the soup into a blender with the coconut milk and 1 cup of the chopped kale and blend until smooth.

Return the soup to the pot and stir in the remaining 2 cups of kale. Season with the salt and simmer until the kale is wilted, another 5 minutes or so. Stir in the cilantro and lime juice and season to taste with fish sauce (or salt) and pepper.

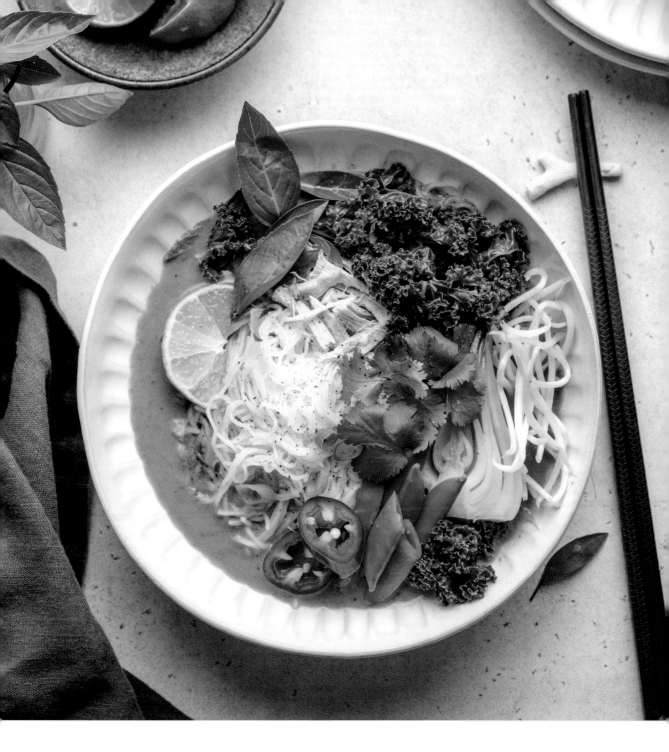

6. Divide the noodles among four bowls. Pour the hot broth into the bowls, dividing it equally among them, then arrange the toppings on the noodles. Serve with lime wedges.

Roasted Tomatillo Tortilla Soup

Yield: 4 servings
Prep Time: 10 minutes
Cook Time: 40 minutes

When it comes to tortilla soup, I can't help but think of my mother-in-law. It's one of her favorite soups. For this version, I marry my favorite roasted tomatillo soup with her tortilla soup—and lo and behold, it's become one of my husband's favorite soups! I guess that's what happens when two good things join forces.

4 medium tomatillos, husked and cleaned

½ cup fresh cilantro leaves, plus more for garnish

1 tablespoon extra-virgin olive oil

1 cup diced yellow onions (about 1 medium onion)

2 cloves garlic, minced

¼ teaspoon kosher salt

4 cups chicken stock

1 teaspoon ground cumin

1 boneless, skinless chicken breast (6 to 8 ounces)

1 (8-inch) flour or corn tortilla, grilled, sliced into thin strips

1 avocado, peeled and sliced into 1-inch chunks

Crème fraîche or sour cream, for serving

1 lime, sliced into wedges, for serving

1. Preheat the oven to 375°F with a rack placed in the center of the oven.

2. Place the tomatillos on a sheet pan and roast for 30 minutes, flipping after 15 minutes. The tomatillos are done when browned and soft to the touch. Let cool for a few minutes, then transfer the tomatillos to a food processor with the cilantro and purée. Set aside.

3. Meanwhile, heat the olive oil in a medium saucepan over medium heat. Add the onions and cook until softened, about 4 minutes. Add the garlic and season with the salt. Add the chicken stock, cumin, and chicken breast and bring to a boil. Lower the heat to a simmer and cook until the chicken is cooked through, about 15 minutes. Remove and shred the chicken. Set aside.

4. Working in batches, put the tomatillo puree and soup in a blender and blend until smooth. Return to the saucepan and heat over medium heat until it returns to a simmer. Adjust the seasoning as necessary, then return the chicken to the pan to heat it through.

5. Serve hot with the tortilla strips, avocado chunks, a dollop of crème fraîche, additional cilantro, and a lime wedge.

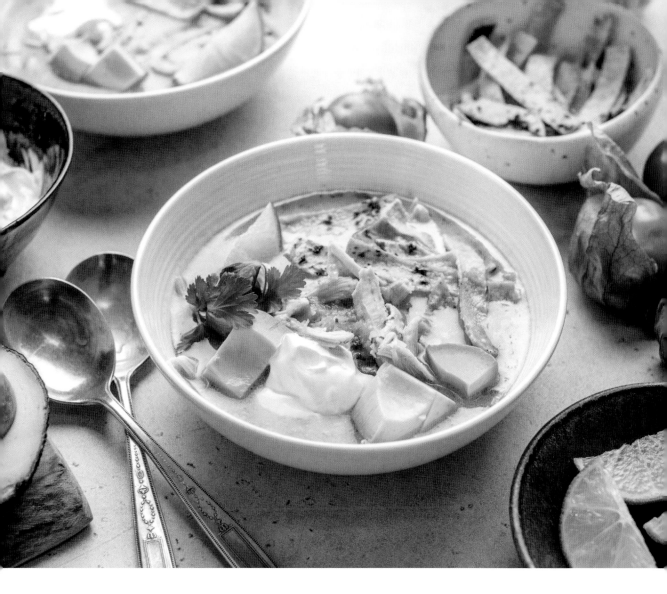

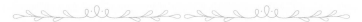

NOTES

When it comes to tortilla strips, there's often a discussion about whether you're on team fried or team soft. I am on team soft, because I like the tortilla strips to function like noodles, and because I am too lazy to fry the tortillas for the team fried members of my family.

For those who prefer the crispy tortilla strips, you can do as my mother-in-law does and replace the flour tortillas with tortilla chips—it's much simpler! Her other shortcut is to use frozen cooked chicken strips and add them to the broth.

Vegetable, Beef, and Barley Soup

Yield: 6 servings

Prep Time: 10 minutes

Cook Time: 1 hour 20 minutes

Beef and barley soup is one of those standards that I feel should be required reading if the kitchen were a library. But I've always felt that it could benefit from more veggies, so I remedy that problem here. The tender beef and hearty barley are balanced with a more generous helping of vegetables and some greens for good measure.

1 cup pearl barley

1 pound stew beef

3 teaspoons kosher salt, divided

¾ teaspoon freshly ground black pepper, divided

½ cup all-purpose flour

3 tablespoons extra-virgin olive oil, divided

1 cup diced yellow onions (about 1 medium onion)

1 clove garlic, minced

1 cup diced carrots (about 2 medium carrots)

1 cup diced celery (about 2 medium stalks)

8 ounces sliced mushrooms (any type)

1 tablespoon tomato paste

7 cups beef stock

1 cup diced butternut squash

1 cup diced zucchini

2 cups baby spinach or chopped kale

1 tablespoon sherry vinegar

1 tablespoon soy sauce

1 teaspoon fresh thyme leaves, plus fresh thyme sprigs for garnish if desired

1. Place the barley in a small bowl, cover with boiling water, and allow to sit for 10 to 15 minutes. Drain, rinse well in a sieve, and set aside.

2. Place the beef in a bowl. Season the meat on all sides with 1 teaspoon of the salt and ½ teaspoon of the pepper. Add the flour and toss to lightly coat the meat on all sides.

3. Heat 2 tablespoons of the olive oil in a Dutch oven or soup pot over medium heat. Working in batches, brown the beef on all sides, then set aside.

4. Heat the remaining tablespoon of oil in the same pot. Sauté the onions until translucent, about 4 minutes. Add the garlic, carrots, celery, and mushrooms and continue to sauté until the mushrooms begin to soften, about 5 minutes. Add the tomato paste, beef stock, and browned beef and season with the remaining 2 teaspoons of salt and ¼ teaspoon of pepper. Bring to a boil, then lower the heat and simmer, partially covered, until the beef is tender, about 30 minutes.

5. Add the softened barley, butternut squash, and zucchini, cover the pot, and cook, stirring occasionally, for another 30 minutes, or until the barley is fully cooked and the squash is fork-tender. Add the spinach and let it wilt. Stir in the vinegar, soy sauce, and thyme leaves. Adjust the seasoning as necessary with salt and pepper. Garnish with thyme sprigs, if desired, and enjoy!

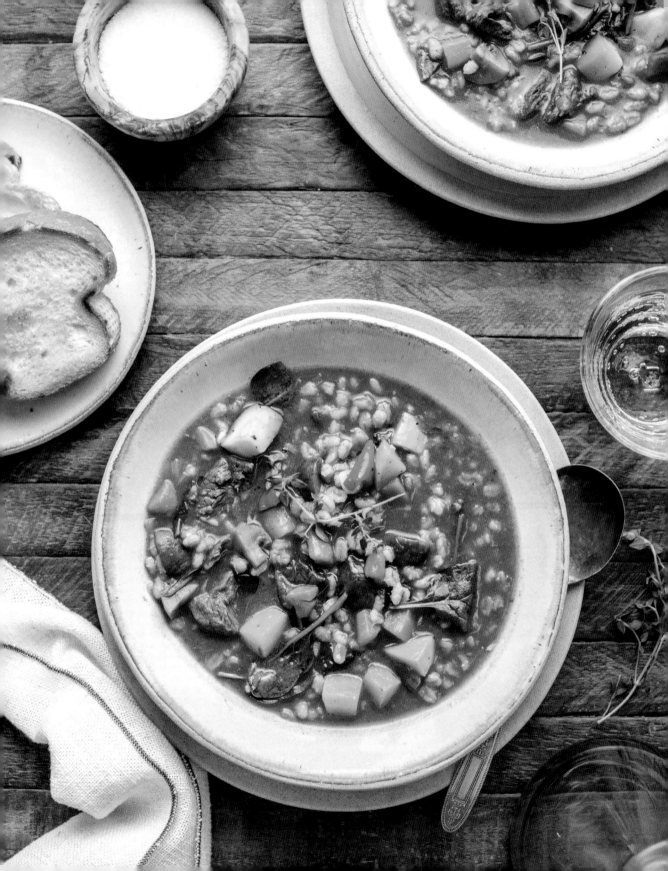

Yield: 6 servings

Prep Time: 15 minutes

Cook Time: 1 hour 10 minutes, or 4 or 8 hours, depending on cooking method used

Kabocha Squash Chili

A bowl of cozy chili is my secret excuse to make cornbread, but I won't deny that the chili is amazing, too! I especially love it on chilly fall evenings, and it's a tradition for our family on Halloween night. Over the years, we transitioned from eating your classic beef chili to vegetarian versions, and this kabocha squash chili is one of them. For the beans, I like to use one can each of kidney, black, cannellini, or pinto beans.

1 tablespoon extra-virgin olive oil

½ cup chopped yellow onions

2 cloves garlic, minced

½ small kabocha squash, peeled, seeded, and cut into ½-inch cubes (about 1 cup)

1 teaspoon soy sauce

1 teaspoon ground cumin

1 teaspoon dried oregano leaves

1 teaspoon paprika

½ teaspoon cayenne pepper

3 (14-ounce) cans beans of choice (ideally a mixture), drained and rinsed

1 (28-ounce) can diced tomatoes

2 cups vegetable stock

5 stalks celery, finely diced

2 to 3 tablespoons granulated sugar

2 tablespoons tomato paste

1 teaspoon Worcestershire sauce

Kosher salt and freshly ground black pepper

SUGGESTED TOPPINGS:

Sliced green onions

Sour cream

Fresh cilantro

Sliced jalapeños

Diced avocado

Finely diced red onions

Crumbled cotija cheese

Cornbread, for serving (optional)

1. In a slow cooker (or a Dutch oven or other large pot), heat the olive oil over medium-low heat. Add the onions, garlic, and squash and season with the soy sauce. Cook until the onions have wilted, 4 to 5 minutes.

2. Add the cumin, oregano, paprika, and cayenne pepper and stir for 30 seconds to coat the squash and give the spices a chance to become fragrant.

3. Stir in the beans, diced tomatoes, vegetable stock, celery, sugar, tomato paste, and Worcestershire sauce. Increase the heat to high, bring to a boil, and then lower the heat to a simmer. The longer the chili cooks, the better it tastes (and I do believe it tastes better the next day). If using a slow cooker, transfer the chili to the slow cooker and let it bubble for 4 hours on high or 8 hours on low. Otherwise, cover and cook for at least an hour, stirring occasionally. Regardless of cooking method, taste the chili often, adjusting the seasoning as necessary with salt and pepper.

4. Use an immersion blender to blend some (but not all) of the chili for a thicker texture.

5. Serve with the toppings of your choice and a slice of cornbread, if desired.

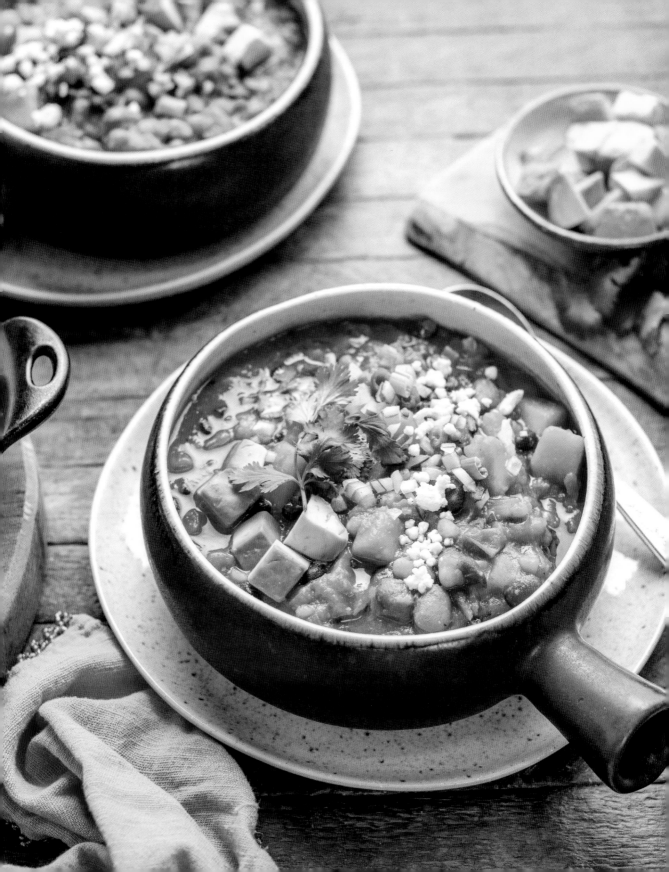

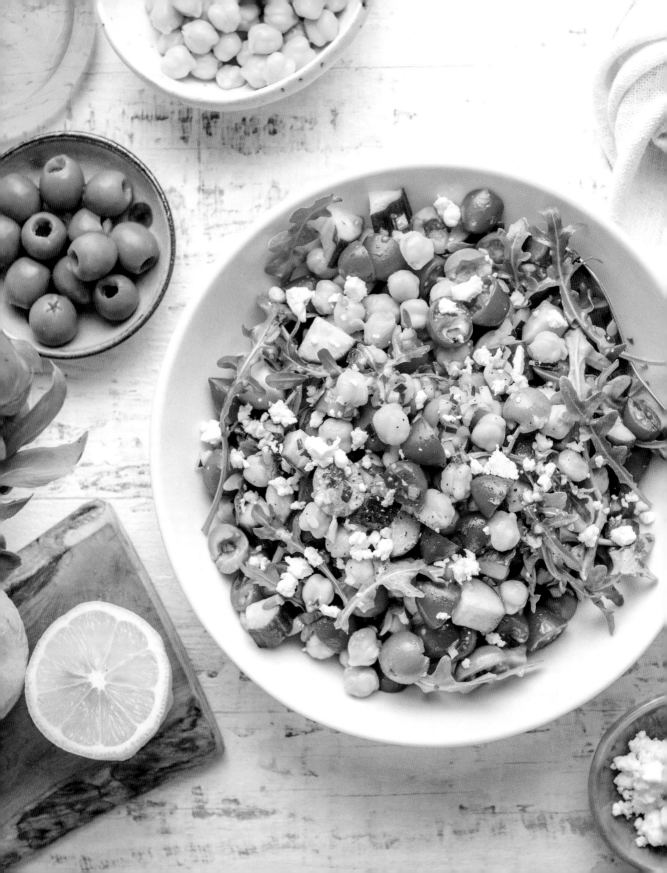

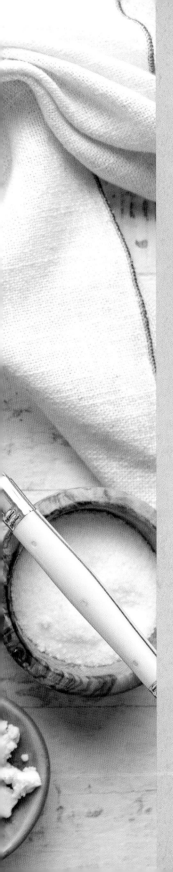

Salads

Grilled Peach Salad *with* Goat Cheese

Yield: 4 to 6 servings
Prep Time: 10 minutes
Cook Time: 5 minutes

When you fire up the grill, be sure to save some grate space for fruit! I just love how grilling the peaches brings out the sweetness even more and softens them up perfectly so they soak in the dressing in this summery salad.

FOR THE DRESSING:

2 tablespoons minced shallot (about 1 small shallot)

1 tablespoon white balsamic vinegar

1 tablespoon fresh lemon juice

3 tablespoons extra-virgin olive oil

Kosher salt and freshly ground black pepper

FOR THE SALAD:

4 ripe but firm peaches, halved, pitted, and sliced into wedges

1 teaspoon extra-virgin olive oil

6 ounces baby kale

⅓ cup crumbled fresh (soft) goat cheese

¼ cup candied walnuts (see Notes)

Kosher salt and freshly ground black pepper

Make the dressing:

1. In a small bowl, cover the shallot with the vinegar and let sit for 5 minutes. Stir in the lemon juice; then, while whisking, drizzle in the olive oil. Season to taste with salt and pepper. Set aside.

Make the salad:

2. Preheat a grill or grill pan to high heat.

3. In a medium bowl, toss the peaches with the olive oil, making sure they are evenly coated on all sides. Grill the peaches for 2 to 3 minutes per side; a fish spatula works really well for flipping the fruit without marring the grill marks.

4. Place the kale, grilled peaches, goat cheese, and candied walnuts in a salad bowl. Give the dressing a quick whisk, then drizzle it over the salad. Toss the salad and season to taste with salt and pepper. Serve immediately.

NOTES

The peaches can be grilled in advance—let them cool completely, then store in an airtight container in the refrigerator for up to 2 days.

Candied walnuts can be made at home, but I love to keep store-bought candied nuts on hand to save time. Trader Joe's sells delicious candied walnuts!

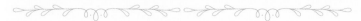

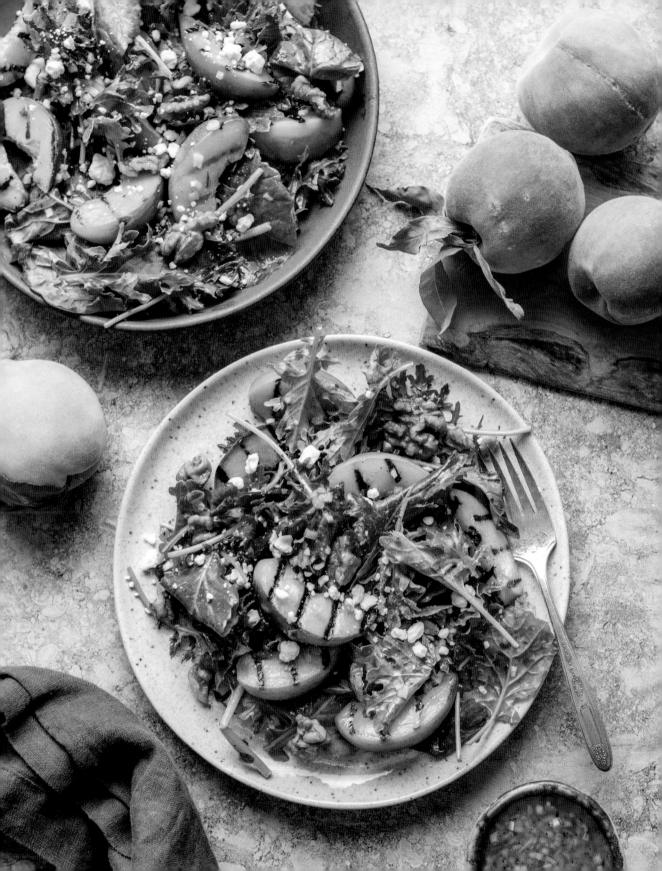

Grilled Fig *and* Halloumi Salad

Yield: 4 to 6 servings
Prep Time: 10 minutes
Cook Time: 5 minutes

If there's one thing I look forward to all summer long, it's fig season. I can't get enough of them, whether they're baked in a galette, eaten simply with a drizzle of honey, or served in a salad like this one. The sweetness of the grilled figs combined with the tanginess of the fig dressing and the saltiness of the squeaky Halloumi cheese is simply magical. If you don't have a grill or grill pan, don't worry—just use a skillet!

FOR THE DRESSING:

2 tablespoons minced shallot (about 1 small shallot)

1 tablespoon balsamic vinegar

1 tablespoon sherry vinegar

4 ripe fresh figs, peeled and mashed

1 teaspoon whole-grain mustard

3 tablespoons extra-virgin olive oil

Kosher salt and freshly ground black pepper

FOR THE SALAD:

1 pound fresh, ripe small figs (about 12), cut in half lengthwise

8 ounces Halloumi cheese, sliced

1 tablespoon extra-virgin olive oil

6 ounces baby greens (see Notes)

½ cup thinly sliced red onions

Make the dressing:

1. In a small bowl, cover the shallot with the balsamic and sherry vinegars and let sit for 5 minutes. Stir in the mashed figs and mustard, then whisk in the olive oil until completely combined. Season to taste with salt and pepper. Set aside.

Make the salad:

2. Preheat a grill or grill pan to high heat.

3. In a medium bowl, toss the halved figs and slices of Halloumi cheese with the olive oil, making sure they are evenly coated on all sides. Grill the figs and cheese for 2 to 3 minutes per side; the cheese should have some grill marks and start to soften and melt.

4. Place the greens on a platter and arrange the grilled figs, cheese, and red onions on top. Give the dressing a quick whisk, then drizzle it over the salad. Serve immediately.

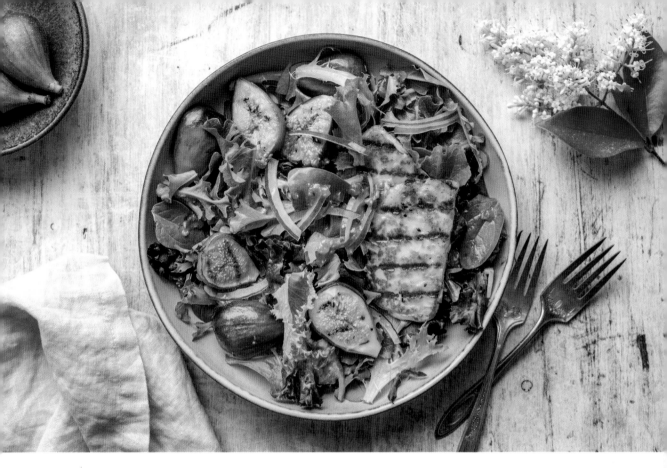

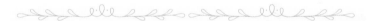

NOTES

The ripeness of the figs is important for this salad. Select figs that are dark in color and soft to the touch; perfectly ripe figs are tender and may even have light wrinkles or stretch marks, all indicators that the figs had ample time to ripen on the tree. If your figs are not quite ripe, or even bland, consider using a drizzle of honey in both the dressing and before grilling the figs to give them more sweetness.

I like to use a combination of baby kale, baby spinach, and baby arugula for this salad, but any mix of tender salad greens will do.

The dressing can be made in advance and stored in an airtight container in the refrigerator for up to 4 days. Let it come to room temperature before serving.

Since you are grilling the cheese, you need to serve this salad immediately; the cheese will harden as it cools. It can be reheated if you wish (I've been known to use the microwave), but ideally, enjoy it right away!

Yield: 6 servings

Prep Time: 10 minutes, plus
1 hour 45 minutes to rehydrate
bulgur and chill salad

Cook Time: 5 minutes

Corn Tabbouleh

When summer gives us sweet corn, one of my favorite salads to showcase those kernels is tabbouleh! Tabbouleh is an herbaceous salad dressed with a simple lemon vinaigrette, and it goes so well with any summer meal.

1 cup fine bulgur wheat

2 ears corn, husks removed

½ cup diced red onions

½ cup diced English cucumbers

½ cup quartered grape tomatoes

3 green onions, finely chopped

½ cup chopped fresh cilantro

¼ cup chopped fresh mint

FOR THE DRESSING:

Juice of 1 large lemon

½ teaspoon white balsamic vinegar (optional)

2 cloves garlic, minced

¼ cup extra-virgin olive oil

¾ teaspoon kosher salt

¾ teaspoon freshly ground black pepper

1. Place the bulgur in a large heatproof bowl and cover with boiling water. Let stand for 30 to 45 minutes, until the bulgur has puffed up. When done, drain the bulgur well and place it back in the bowl to cool.

2. Meanwhile, cook the corn: Bring a pot of water to a rolling boil over high heat. Add the ears of corn and cook for 4 to 5 minutes, or until the kernels are a brilliant yellow and just tender and juicy. Drain the corn. When it is cool enough to handle, cut the kernels off the cobs; you should have about 1½ cups of cooked corn kernels.

3. Once the bulgur is cool, add the corn, red onions, cucumbers, tomatoes, green onions, cilantro, and mint to the bowl and give the salad a good stir.

4. Make the dressing: In a small bowl, whisk together the lemon juice, vinegar (if using), garlic, and olive oil and season with the salt and pepper.

5. Add the dressing to the salad and stir until evenly coated. Adjust the seasoning with salt and pepper if necessary. Chill the salad in the refrigerator for 30 minutes to an hour before serving. Keep in a tightly sealed container in the refrigerator until ready to serve.

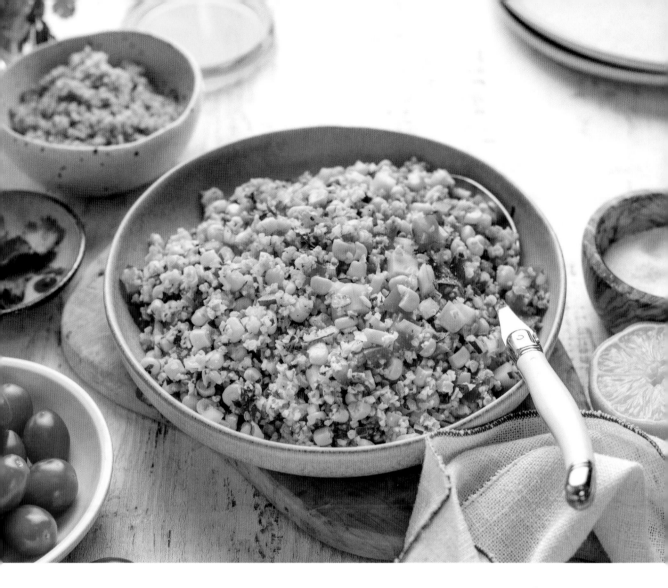

NOTES

Corn tabbouleh lasts for up to 3 days when stored in the refrigerator. The flavors taste better the longer it sits.

While white balsamic vinegar is not traditional in tabbouleh, I find that adding a touch of it helps to balance the acidity of the dish. The natural sweetness in balsamic vinegar works well with the lemon juice, rounding out the flavors of the salad.

A traditional tabbouleh uses flat-leaf parsley, but I prefer cilantro in this version for its citrus notes and mellow flavor. I also love how it pairs with summer corn and tomatoes.

Brussels Sprouts Caesar Salad

Yield: 4 to 6 servings

Prep Time: 10 minutes

Caesar salad is a favorite at our house and makes a weekly appearance. But once in a while, I like to swap out the romaine for nutrient-packed Brussels sprouts! It's a great way to add fiber and antioxidants to a classic salad that I know the family will love.

2 cloves garlic, minced

1 teaspoon anchovy paste

1 teaspoon kosher salt

Pinch of freshly ground black pepper

1 tablespoon fresh lemon juice

1 teaspoon Worcestershire sauce

½ teaspoon Dijon mustard

½ cup mayonnaise

1 (16-ounce) bag shaved Brussels sprouts

1 cup croutons

2 ounces bacon, cooked and crumbled (optional)

1¼ cups grated Parmigiano-Reggiano cheese, or ½ cup shaved with a vegetable peeler

1. In a large salad bowl, mash the garlic, anchovy paste, salt, and pepper with a fork until you have a paste. Whisk in the lemon juice, Worcestershire sauce, mustard, and mayonnaise. Season to taste with additional salt and pepper if necessary.

2. Add the Brussels sprouts, croutons, bacon (if using), and cheese and toss to combine.

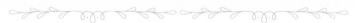

NOTES

You can usually find shaved Brussels sprouts in the produce department; if not, you can thinly slice 1 pound of whole sprouts in a food processor using the slicing attachment. Or, of course, you can simply use a knife!

If slicing whole Brussels sprouts, try to use smaller, younger ones, which are usually sweeter. Brussels sprouts can sometimes be bitter, especially when older or larger. Also, a little time in the dressing (about 15 minutes) helps to balance the flavor. If you find that the flavor of your sprouts would benefit from some resting time after dressing, be sure to wait until right before serving to add the croutons to the salad so they stay nice and crunchy.

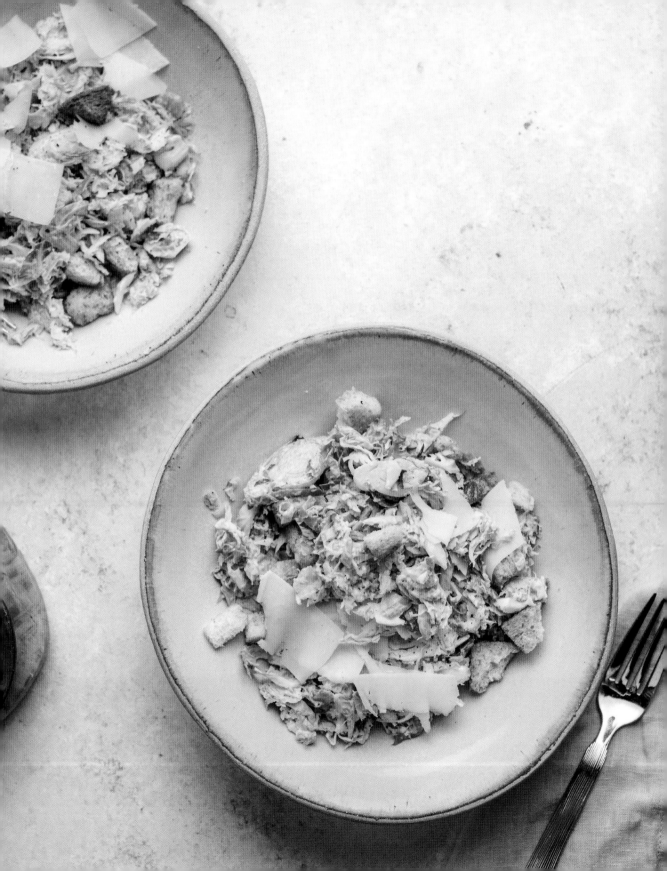

Chickpea Summer Salad

Yield: 4 to 6 servings

Prep Time: 10 minutes, plus 1 hour to chill

This salad has long been a staple at our house—it is my go-to summer side dish, the one that goes with practically every meal! I have different varieties, and this one in particular celebrates everything I love about Mediterranean flavors, with briny olives, tangy feta cheese, and beautiful summer tomatoes.

1 (15-ounce) can chickpeas

1½ cups diced English cucumber

1½ cups halved grape tomatoes

½ cup finely diced red onions

½ cup halved olives (such as Castelvetrano, Kalamata, or Niçoise)

⅓ cup minced fresh cilantro

3 tablespoons torn fresh basil leaves

2 cloves garlic, minced

1 teaspoon salt

3 tablespoons extra-virgin olive oil

2 tablespoons fresh lemon juice

2 teaspoons white wine vinegar

1 teaspoon Dijon mustard

Freshly ground black pepper

1 cup arugula

¼ cup crumbled feta cheese

1. Rinse and drain the chickpeas.

2. In a medium bowl, combine the chickpeas, cucumber, tomatoes, red onions, olives, and herbs.

3. In a small bowl, mash the garlic and salt with a fork. Whisk in the olive oil, lemon juice, vinegar, and mustard. Season to taste with pepper.

4. Pour the dressing over the salad and toss to coat. Let sit in the refrigerator for at least an hour.

5. Right before serving, stir in the arugula and feta cheese.

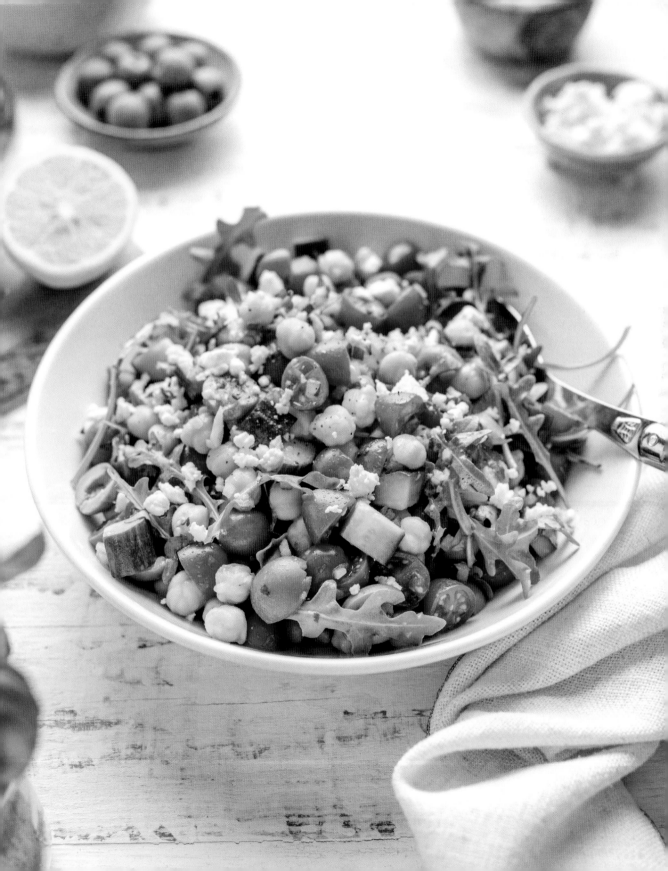

Yield: 6 servings

Prep Time: 15 minutes

Cook Time: 15 minutes

Flank Steak *and* Artichoke Salad

If you forced me to pick one cut of meat to cook forever, it would have to be flank steak. It's lean yet flavorful, affordable, and extremely versatile, perfect for grilling, roasting, or sautéing! I especially love it grilled and enjoyed in a salad, and this one pops with marinated artichokes, peppers, and onions—it's delicious any time of year.

FOR THE DRESSING:

⅓ cup extra-virgin olive oil

2 tablespoons balsamic vinegar

1 teaspoon Dijon mustard

1 teaspoon minced garlic

1 teaspoon honey

Kosher salt and freshly ground black pepper

FOR THE RUB:

1½ tablespoons kosher salt

1 tablespoon garlic powder

½ teaspoon freshly ground black pepper

½ teaspoon ground white pepper

¼ teaspoon cayenne pepper

¼ teaspoon onion powder

FOR THE SALAD:

1¼ pounds flank steak

12 ounces arugula

2 cups spinach

1 cup thinly sliced red onions (about 1 medium onion)

1 cup marinated quartered artichokes

1 cup sliced roasted red peppers

½ cup halved cherry tomatoes

Kosher salt and freshly ground black pepper

2 tablespoons crumbled feta cheese

¼ cup pea shoots (optional)

Make the dressing:

1. Place the olive oil, vinegar, mustard, garlic, and honey in a jar. Season to taste with salt and pepper. Seal the lid and shake vigorously. (You can also do this with a bowl and a whisk.) Set aside.

Make the rub and season the steak:

2. In a small bowl, mix together the salt, garlic powder, peppers, and onion powder. Generously season the steak on both sides with the rub and let it sit at room temperature while the grill heats up.

Grill the steak and make the salad:

3. Preheat a grill or grill pan to medium-high heat. Grill the steak for about 6 minutes per side, until a thermometer inserted into the thickest part reads 120°F to 125°F for rare, 130°F to 140°F for medium-rare, or 145°F for medium. Allow the steak to rest on a cutting board while you prepare the rest of the salad.

4. In a large bowl, toss together the greens, red onions, artichokes, roasted red peppers, and tomatoes.

5. Lightly dress the salad with some of the dressing, season to taste with salt and pepper, and then arrange on a platter. Slice the steak against the grain and place on top of the salad. Drizzle with a little more dressing and top with the feta cheese and pea shoots, if using.

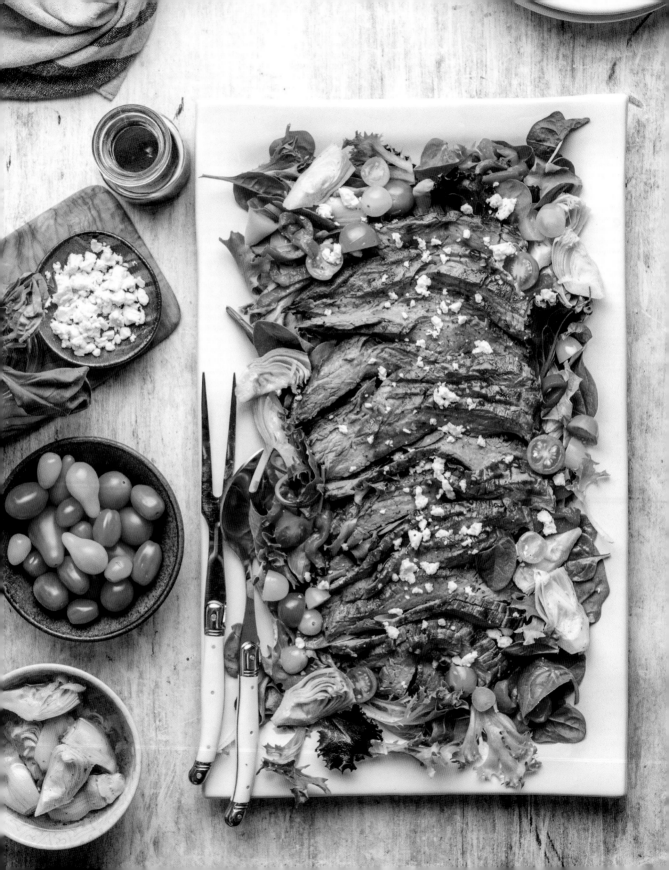

Little Gem Salad *with* Apple *and* Beets

Yield: 4 servings

Prep Time: 10 minutes

My mom used to make a delicious Russian beet potato salad, and my favorite part was the crunchy apples. I couldn't help but think of it when I made this salad, with its creamy dressing, juicy apples, and earthy beets! It's a simple salad that is especially lovely in the fall when apples are sweet and plentiful.

FOR THE DRESSING:

¼ cup chopped fresh dill, plus extra for garnish if desired

3 tablespoons extra-virgin olive oil

2 tablespoons white wine vinegar

1 teaspoon anchovy paste

½ cup sour cream

Kosher salt and freshly ground black pepper

FOR THE SALAD:

5 ounces little gems or butter lettuce

1 apple, such as Honeycrisp or Fuji, sliced

3 beets, cooked, peeled, and sliced

¼ cup thinly sliced red onions

Kosher salt and freshly ground black pepper

1. Make the dressing: Place the dill, olive oil, vinegar, and anchovy paste in a food processor. Process on high speed to combine. Add the sour cream and pulse until the dressing is blended. Season to taste with salt and pepper.

2. Toss the lettuce with half of the dressing until fully coated. Stir in the apple, beets, red onions, and more dressing, as needed, to dress the salad. Season to taste with salt and pepper. Garnish with more dill, if desired, and enjoy immediately.

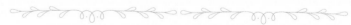

NOTES

I like to keep a tube of anchovy paste in the refrigerator—it's a handy way to add punch to a dish, and it's easy to sneak in when you've got people who aren't fans of anchovies in the house. If you're wary, don't fret; anchovy paste adds a nice saltiness—think Caesar salad dressing. If you prefer to use canned anchovies, replace the paste with 2 anchovy fillets and mash them with a fork before using in the recipe.

To save time, store-bought precooked beets make this salad a cinch to throw together!

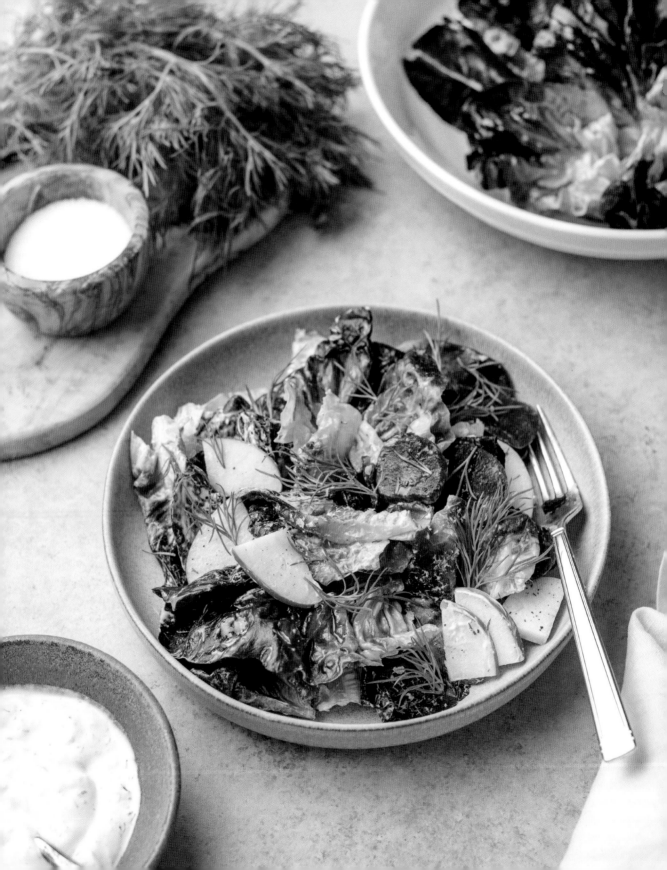

Yield: 6 servings

Prep Time: 15 minutes, plus 30 minutes to rest kale

Cook Time: 20 minutes

Kale Quinoa Salad
with Grapes

Grapes often get overlooked when it comes to recipes, which is truly a shame, because they can lend sweetness, juiciness, and texture to sweet and savory dishes! This kale salad is one of my favorites, with bursts of brightness from the plump grapes, crunch from the walnuts, and satisfying, protein-rich quinoa.

FOR THE SALAD:

1 tablespoon extra-virgin olive oil

Kosher salt

1 pound curly kale, destemmed and chopped (about 6 cups)

1 cup quinoa

2 cups water

2 cups halved red grapes

½ cup crumbled feta cheese

½ cup chopped roasted walnuts

Freshly ground black pepper

FOR THE DRESSING:

1 medium shallot, minced (about ⅓ cup)

2 tablespoons sherry vinegar

1 tablespoon fresh lemon juice

1 teaspoon Dijon mustard

1 teaspoon honey

½ cup plus 1 tablespoon extra-virgin olive oil

Kosher salt and freshly ground black pepper

Prepare the kale:

1. In a large bowl, massage the olive oil and ½ teaspoon of salt into the kale with your hands for 1 minute. The kale will shrink in volume. Let sit at room temperature for 30 minutes while you prepare the other components.

Prepare the quinoa:

2. Rinse and drain the quinoa in a sieve. Combine the quinoa and water in a 2-quart saucepan and bring to a boil over medium-high heat. Lower the heat to a simmer, cover the pan, and cook for about 15 minutes, until the liquid is absorbed. Remove the pan from the heat and let the quinoa steam, covered, for about 5 minutes. Transfer the quinoa to a sheet pan, spread it out, and let cool until no longer hot, then place in the refrigerator until fully cool.

Make the dressing:

3. In a small bowl, whisk together the shallot, vinegar, lemon juice, mustard, and honey. While whisking, slowly pour in the olive oil. Season to taste with salt and pepper.

Make the salad:

4. Add the cooked quinoa, grapes, and half of the dressing to the kale and toss well to combine. Stir in the feta cheese and walnuts and season to taste with salt and pepper, adding more dressing if desired.

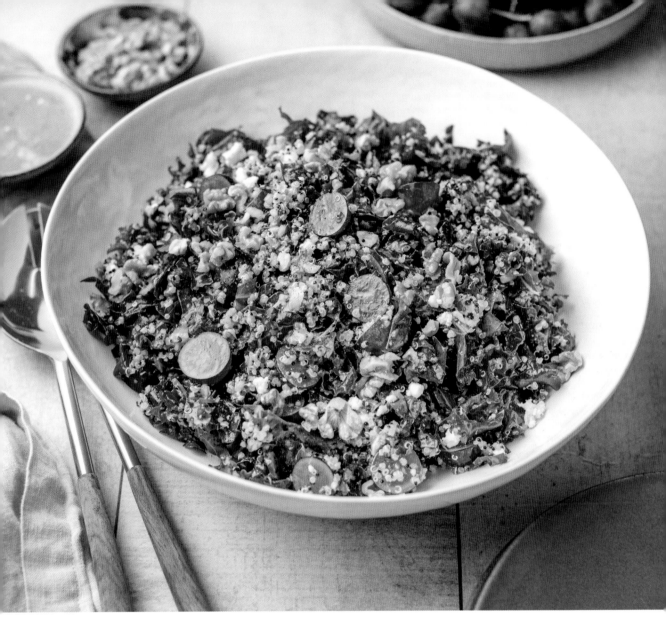

NOTE

Because of the kale, this salad is sturdy enough to make in advance or enjoy left over. You can massage the kale and prep the components a day in advance, then toss when ready to serve. Alternatively, you can simply toss everything together, including the dressing, and store it in a tightly sealed container in the refrigerator until ready to serve, or up to 4 days.

Winter Squash Quinoa Salad

Yield: 6 servings

Prep Time: 15 minutes, plus 30 minutes to rest kale

Cook Time: 25 minutes

This wintry version of a quinoa salad is the perfect way to highlight your favorite fall squashes. I use butternut squash, but it is also delicious with roasted acorn squash or delicata squash! It is a hearty salad that can take you from autumn to winter, and it's perfect for Thanksgiving dinner or any weeknight meal.

FOR THE SALAD:

1 medium butternut squash, peeled, seeded, and cut into 1-inch cubes

3 tablespoons extra-virgin olive oil, divided

Kosher salt and freshly ground black pepper

1 pound curly kale, destemmed and chopped (about 6 cups)

1 cup quinoa

2 cups water

½ cup roasted and salted shelled pumpkin seeds

½ cup sweetened dried cranberries

⅓ cup crumbled fresh (soft) goat cheese

FOR THE DRESSING:

1 medium shallot, minced (about ⅓ cup)

3 tablespoons white balsamic vinegar

1 teaspoon Dijon mustard

1 teaspoon honey

½ cup plus 1 tablespoon extra-virgin olive oil

Kosher salt and freshly ground black pepper

Roast the squash:

1. Preheat the oven to 400°F with a rack placed in the center of the oven.

2. Place the butternut squash on a sheet pan, drizzle with 2 tablespoons of the olive oil, season generously with salt and pepper, and toss well, using your hands to evenly coat the squash. Spread out the squash and roast for 15 to 20 minutes, or until fork-tender.

Prepare the kale:

3. In a large bowl, use your hands to massage the remaining tablespoon of olive oil and ½ teaspoon of salt into the kale for 1 minute. The kale will shrink in volume. Let sit at room temperature for 30 minutes while you prepare the other components.

Prepare the quinoa:

4. Rinse and drain the quinoa in a sieve. Combine the quinoa and water in a 2-quart saucepan and bring to a boil over medium-high heat. Lower the heat to a simmer, cover the pan, and cook for about 15 minutes, until the liquid is absorbed. Remove from the heat and let the quinoa steam, covered, for about 5 minutes. Transfer the quinoa to a sheet pan, spread it out, and let cool until no longer hot, then place in the refrigerator until fully cool.

Make the dressing:

5. In a small bowl, whisk together the shallot, vinegar, mustard, and honey. While whisking, slowly pour in the olive oil. Season to taste with salt and pepper. Set the dressing aside or refrigerate it until you are ready to assemble the salad.

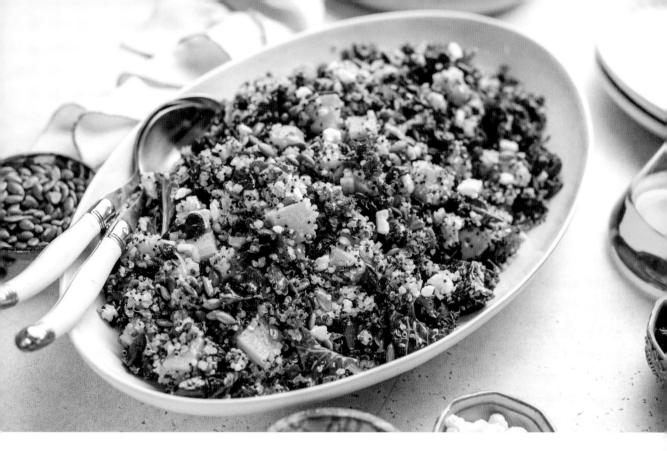

Make the salad:

6. Add the quinoa, roasted squash, and half of the dressing to the kale and toss well. Stir in the pumpkin seeds, cranberries, and goat cheese and season to taste with salt and pepper, adding more dressing if desired.

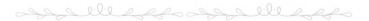

NOTES

This salad may have a number of components, but they all can be prepared simultaneously or, even better, in advance. Because this is a pretty large and hearty salad that keeps well, I like to make it at the beginning of the week and serve it for lunch or dinner throughout the week.

The kale can be massaged and the components prepped up to a day in advance, then tossed when ready to serve. If you prefer to prep the whole salad in advance, toss everything together, including the dressing, and store in a tightly sealed container in the refrigerator until ready to serve, or up to 4 days.

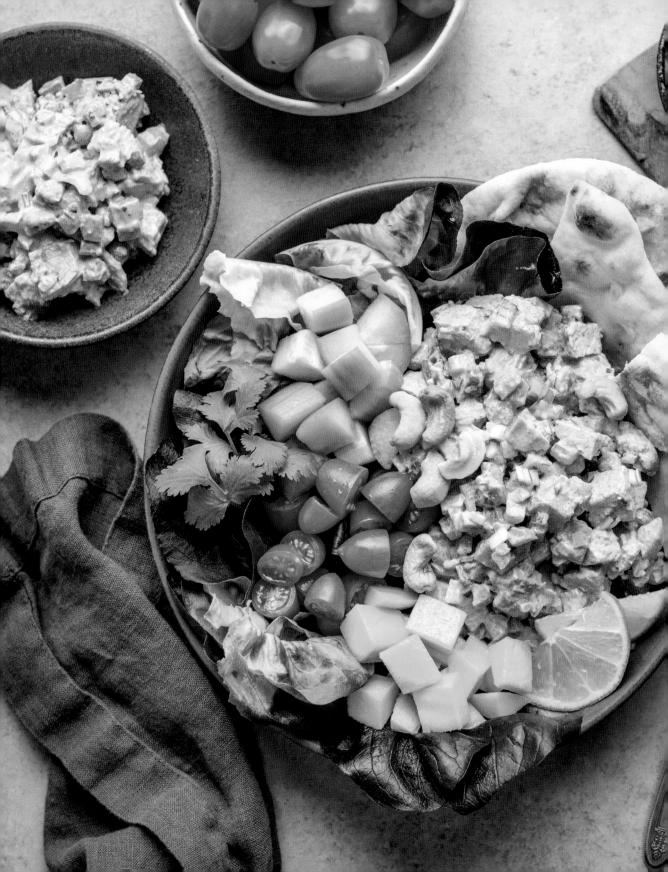

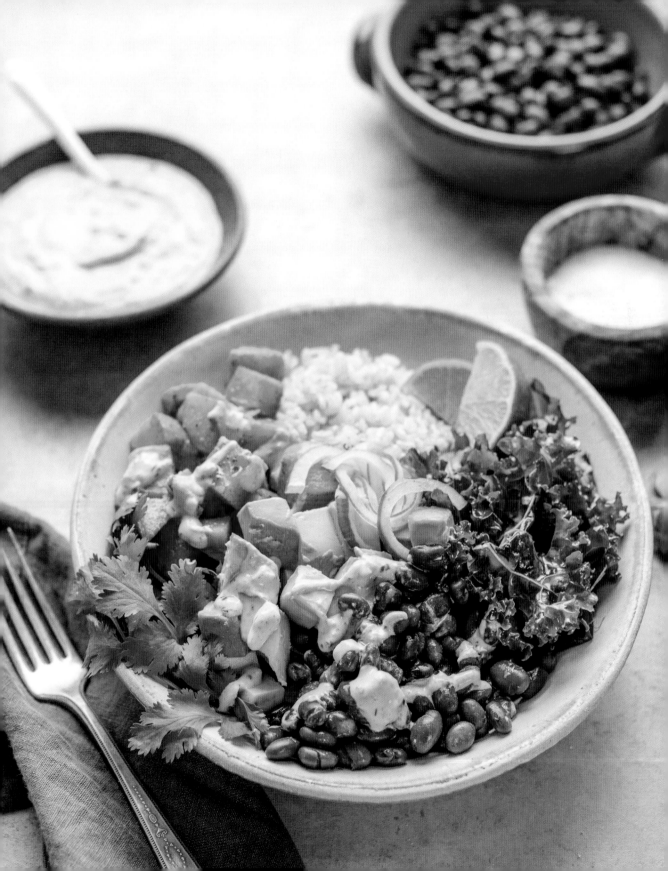

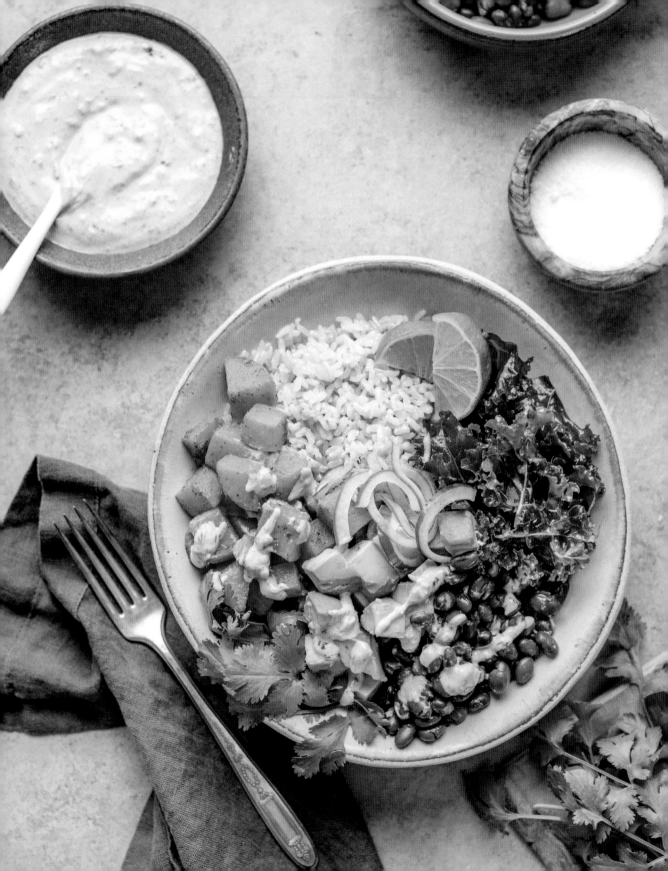

coriander, and garlic powder. Sprinkle the spice blend onto the sweet potatoes and toss to evenly coat. Scatter the sweet potatoes on a sheet pan and roast for 15 to 20 minutes, flipping once halfway through, until browned and fork-tender.

5. When the sweet potatoes are fully cooked, transfer to a bowl and toss in the remaining 2 tablespoons of oil.

Make the creamy chipotle sauce:

6. Place the yogurt, chipotle pepper, lime juice, garlic cloves, and a pinch of salt in a blender or small food processor. Blend or process until smooth. Season to taste with salt. Set aside until ready to assemble the bowls, or store in the refrigerator. The sauce can be made a day ahead.

Assemble the bowls:

7. Fill serving bowls with the kale, roasted sweet potatoes, black beans, brown rice, and avocado. Garnish with the pickled red onions, creamy chipotle sauce, and cilantro. Serve with lime wedges.

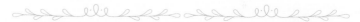

NOTES

Chipotle peppers can be very spicy—if you prefer a milder sauce, start with half a pepper and build to taste. Or, if you're very sensitive to spice, use just a few drops of the canned adobo sauce in place of the chipotle pepper itself.

Similarly, 1 teaspoon of chipotle powder for the sweet potatoes gives them a medium level of spiciness. If you are sensitive to spiciness, use less, to taste, and of course, if you prefer more kick, use more!

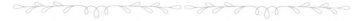

Adobo Meatball Bowls

Yield: 4 servings
Prep Time: 25 minutes
Cook Time: 25 minutes

When you think of Filipino adobo, the first thing to come to mind is chicken or pork, but I love to give an adobo twist to other dishes as well. These adobo meatball bowls take the flavors of my family's classic adobo recipe and put them in delicious meatballs. I garnish them with a quick pickle inspired by achara, a delicious green papaya relish. This version is made even simpler with easy-to-find jicama for extra crunch, which balances the bowls beautifully.

FOR THE QUICK-PICKLED "ACHARA":

(Makes 1½ cups)

½ cup peeled and julienned jicama

1 clove garlic, thinly sliced

1 (1-inch) piece fresh ginger, peeled and julienned

½ cup peeled and julienned carrots

½ cup julienned red bell peppers

½ cup thinly sliced red onions

1 teaspoon thinly sliced Fresno chili

½ cup unseasoned rice vinegar

1 teaspoon granulated sugar

1 teaspoon kosher salt

FOR THE ADOBO MEATBALLS:

1 pound ground pork

½ cup panko breadcrumbs

2 green onions, minced

3 cloves garlic, minced

2 tablespoons soy sauce

2 teaspoons apple cider vinegar

1 large egg, lightly beaten

½ teaspoon kosher salt

½ teaspoon black pepper

2 tablespoons extra-virgin olive oil, for the pan

FOR THE ADOBO GLAZE:

¼ cup honey

¼ cup apple cider vinegar

¼ cup soy sauce

4 cloves garlic, smashed with the side of a knife

1 bay leaf

FOR THE BOWLS:

4 cups cooked brown rice

4 baby broccoli (aka broccolini), or florets from 1 small head regular broccoli, blanched or steamed

1 cup green onion microgreens, or ¼ cup sliced green onions

Handful of fresh cilantro leaves

Black and/or white sesame seeds, for garnish

Sriracha sauce, for garnish (optional)

Make the quick-pickled "achara":

1. Place the jicama, garlic, ginger, carrots, bell peppers, red onions, and Fresno chili in a bowl. In a separate small bowl, whisk together the vinegar, sugar, and salt until the sugar and salt have dissolved. Mix into the vegetables and let sit while you prepare the rest of the dish.

Make the meatballs:

2. Preheat the oven to 350°F with a rack placed in the center of the oven.

(recipe continues on page 157)

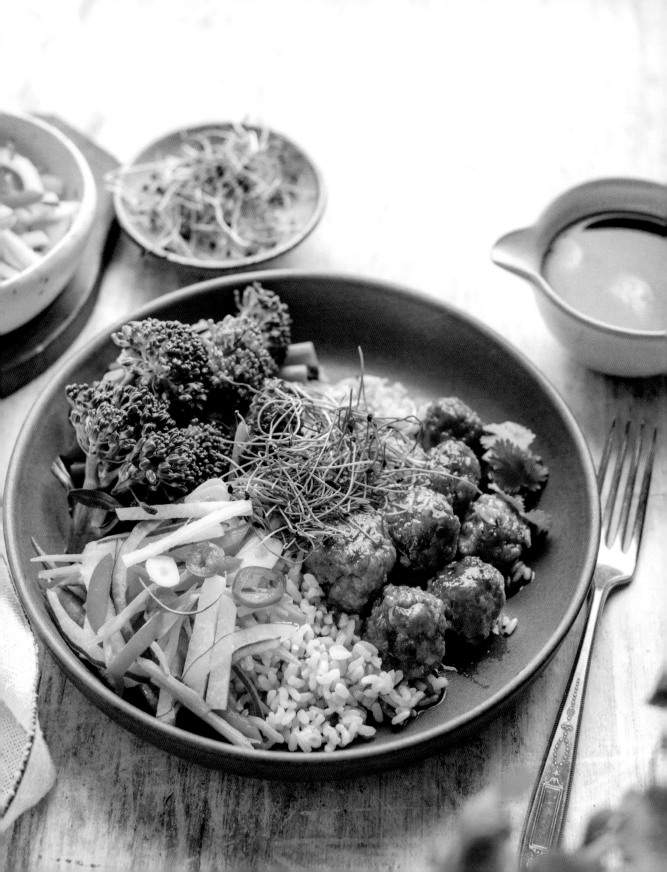

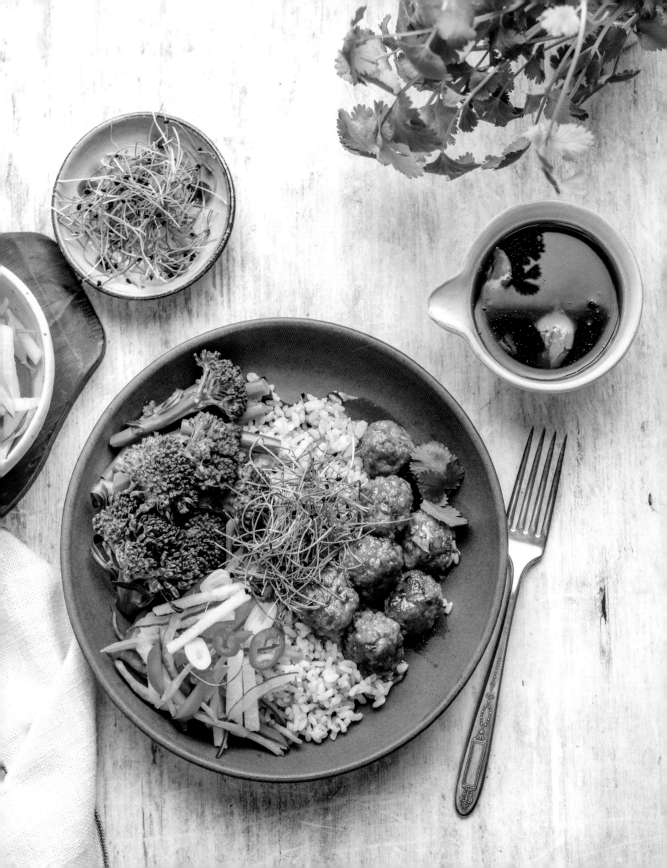

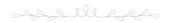

NOTES

This recipe makes more quick-pickled achara than you will need for this dish, but it will keep for a few days and is a great condiment to add to other dishes. Store it in a tightly covered glass container in the refrigerator. It's also a great component to make ahead of time.

The meatballs can also be made in advance—you could either form and store them in a single layer on a covered sheet pan in the refrigerator overnight before cooking, or cook and glaze the meatballs and store in an airtight container in the refrigerator. They can be reheated in a skillet over medium-low heat for about 10 minutes before serving.

Baby broccoli, also known as broccolini or broccolette, is a hybrid of broccoli and Chinese broccoli (gai lan), with longer, thinner stems and a milder, sweeter taste. If you can't find baby broccoli, regular broccoli works just as well in this recipe.

If you can't find Fresno chilis, jalapeño peppers are a good substitute with a similar heat level. However, if you prefer more spice and have access to Thai bird chilis, they work beautifully here, too.

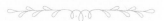

3. In a large bowl, combine the ground pork with the breadcrumbs, green onions, garlic, soy sauce, vinegar, egg, salt, and pepper. Use your hands to form the mixture into meatballs about 1½ inches in diameter; you should get 28 to 30 meatballs.

4. In a sauté pan, heat the olive oil over medium heat. Working in batches, brown the meatballs on all sides, then transfer them to a sheet pan.

5. Bake the meatballs for 10 to 12 minutes, or until cooked through. When done, they will have reached an internal temperature of 160°F.

While the meatballs are cooking, make the glaze:

6. In a small saucepan, stir together the honey, vinegar, soy sauce, garlic, and bay leaf. Place over medium heat and cook for about 5 minutes, until glossy.

7. When the meatballs are ready, remove from the oven and drizzle with enough glaze to coat the meatballs on all sides. Reserve any remaining glaze for serving.

Assemble the bowls:

8. Serve the meatballs over the rice along with the broccoli and quick-pickled achara. Top with the green onion microgreens, cilantro, a sprinkling of sesame seeds, and a drizzle of extra glaze. Finish with a squirt of Sriracha sauce, if desired.

Curry Chicken Salad Bowls

Yield: 4 servings

Prep Time: 10 minutes

I still remember the chicken salad sandwiches my mother used to pack in my lunches when I was a little girl. They were so simple, and they always brought a smile to my face. But when I started making them for myself, I found myself tweaking her base recipe to give the chicken salad more pizzazz. These curry chicken salad bowls take basic chicken salad to the next level, with Greek yogurt to lighten it up, and just the right amount of heat, crunch, and zing! Eating it bowl style makes it easy to add extra veggies!

Meat from 2 roasted chicken breasts, diced

⅓ cup finely diced red onions

⅓ cup chopped fresh chives

⅓ cup finely diced celery

¼ cup golden raisins

¼ cup chopped roasted, salted cashews, plus whole cashews for garnish if desired

½ cup plain Greek yogurt

1 tablespoon curry powder

⅛ teaspoon cayenne pepper

Juice of ½ lime

½ teaspoon kosher salt

Freshly ground black pepper

4 cups lettuce

1 cup diced cucumbers

1 cup halved grape tomatoes

1 mango, pitted, peeled, and diced

4 naan, toasted and cut into wedges

Lime wedges, for serving (optional)

Fresh cilantro leaves, for garnish (optional)

1. In a large bowl, combine the chicken, red onions, chives, celery, raisins, and cashews.

2. In a small bowl, whisk together the yogurt, curry powder, cayenne pepper, and lime juice. Stir the dressing into the chicken mixture until combined. Season with the salt and pepper to taste.

3. Serve the chicken salad on top of the lettuce along with the cucumbers, tomatoes, mango, and toasted naan. If desired, serve with lime wedges and a garnish of cilantro.

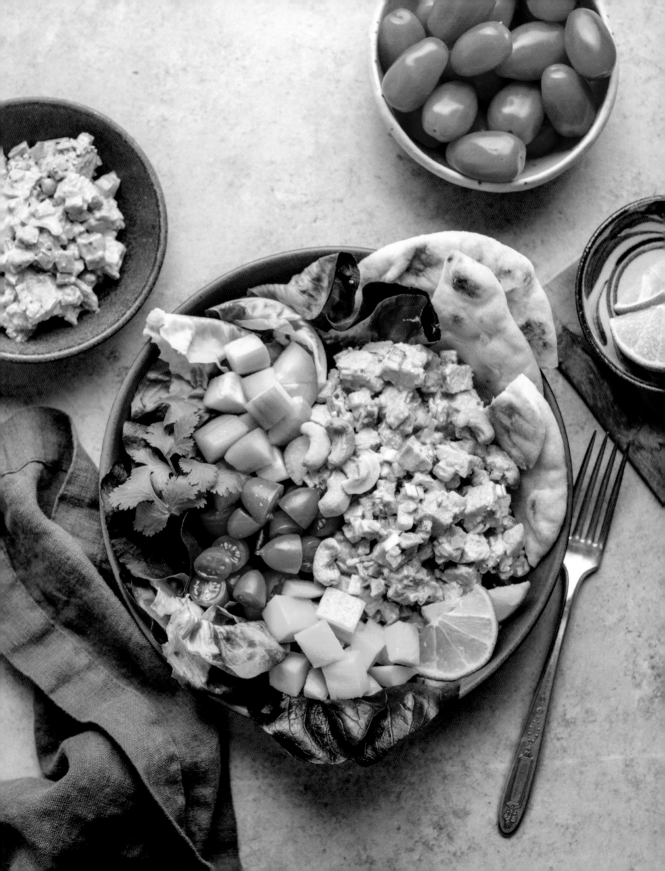

Beef Satay Bowls *with* Cucumber *and* Carrot Slaw

Yield: 4 servings

Prep Time: 20 minutes, plus 1 hour to marinate beef

Cook Time: 10 minutes

Food is always more fun when it's served on a stick, but to be honest, the skewers are optional in these beef satay bowls. An umami-packed marinade imparts Thai-style flavor to sirloin steak, which grills in just minutes and is served up in a bowl packed with a crunchy cucumber and carrot slaw, edamame, and a drizzle of a peanut sauce. This bowl will quickly become a family favorite. I know it is in mine!

FOR THE MARINATED BEEF:

¼ cup honey

¼ cup fish sauce

4 cloves garlic, minced

2 tablespoons soy sauce

2 tablespoons extra-virgin olive oil, plus more to oil grill grates

2 teaspoons grated fresh ginger

1 teaspoon Sriracha sauce

1 teaspoon ground coriander

½ teaspoon turmeric powder

2 tablespoons minced red onions

1 (1-inch) piece lemongrass (from bottom third of stalk), pounded with the flat of the blade of a chef's knife and minced

1¼ pounds top sirloin steak, sliced into 2-inch pieces, ¼ inch thick

SPECIAL EQUIPMENT:

8 (9-inch) wooden or stainless-steel skewers (optional)

FOR THE CUCUMBER AND CARROT SLAW:

1 medium cucumber, cut into 1-inch pieces (about 1½ cups)

1 cup shredded carrots (about 2 medium carrots)

⅓ cup thinly sliced red onions

⅓ cup thinly sliced red bell peppers

1½ cups water

2 teaspoons kosher salt

½ teaspoon granulated sugar

FOR THE PEANUT SAUCE:

¼ cup creamy, salted peanut butter

1 clove garlic, minced

1 tablespoon soy sauce

1 tablespoon lime juice

2 teaspoons Sriracha sauce

1 teaspoon fish sauce

1 teaspoon honey

1 teaspoon untoasted sesame oil (unrefined)

Up to ½ cup boiling water

FOR SERVING/GARNISH:

2 cups cooked brown rice

3 cups fresh or frozen edamame, cooked and shelled

1 cup shredded red cabbage (optional)

Black and/or white sesame seeds, for garnish

Fresh cilantro leaves, for garnish

Lime wedges, for serving

(recipe continues on page 163)

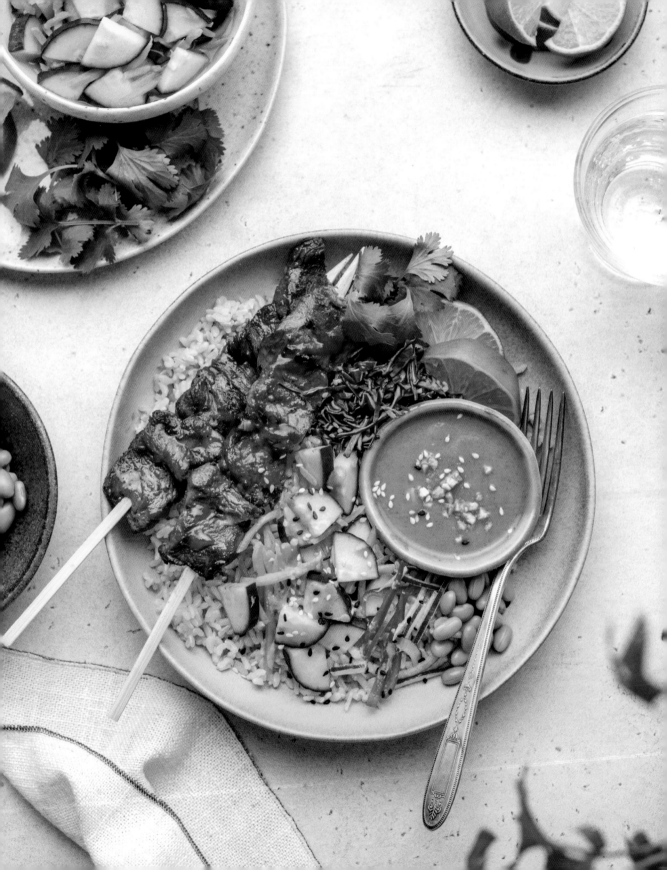

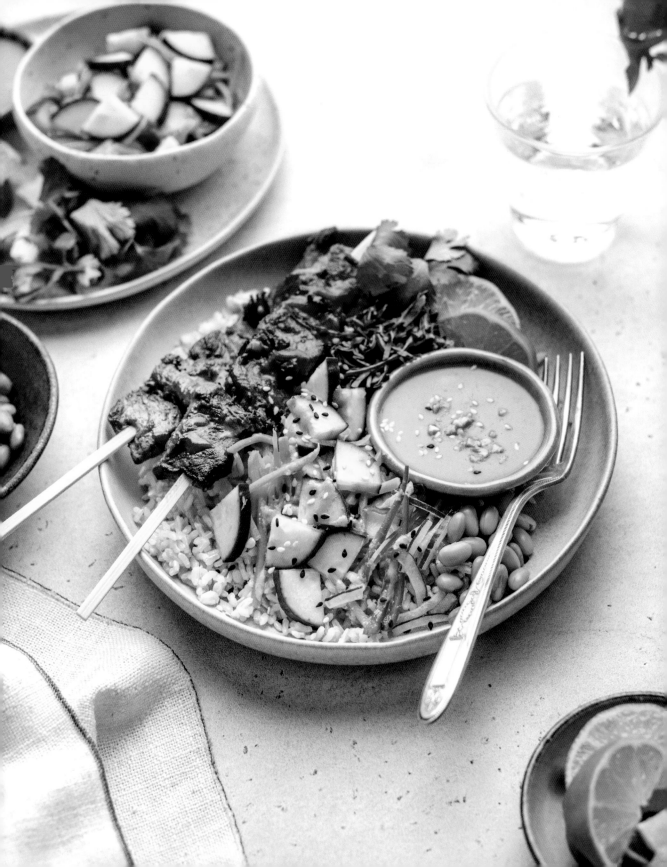

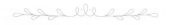

NOTES

Pressed for time? Skip the step of skewering and use a grill pan! You can also cook the beef in a cast-iron skillet; just be sure to work in batches if necessary.

You can also buy preshelled edamame to save yourself a step. For this recipe, you will need 1¼ cups of shelled edamame, fresh or frozen.

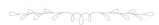

Marinate the beef:

1. In a medium bowl, whisk together the honey, fish sauce, garlic, soy sauce, olive oil, ginger, Sriracha, coriander, and turmeric. Stir in the red onions, lemongrass, and beef, coating well with the marinade. Cover the bowl with plastic wrap and place in the refrigerator for at least 1 hour or overnight.

Make the slaw:

2. In a glass bowl, combine all the ingredients for the slaw, stirring until the salt and sugar have dissolved. Cover and refrigerate until ready to assemble the bowls. The slaw can be made a day in advance.

Cook the beef and assemble the bowls:

3. If using wooden skewers and a grill, soak the skewers in water for at least 30 minutes before grilling. You can also use stainless-steel skewers. Skewer the meat. Alternatively, you can use an outdoor or stovetop grill pan and skip the skewering altogether.

4. Preheat a grill or grill pan to high heat. Lightly oil the grates. Grill the beef for 4 to 5 minutes, turning periodically, until browned. Transfer to a plate to rest.

Make the peanut sauce and assemble the bowls:

5. In a small bowl, whisk together the peanut butter, garlic, soy sauce, lime juice, Sriracha, fish sauce, honey, and sesame oil while slowly drizzling in the hot water until you achieve your desired consistency.

6. Distribute the rice among four bowls. Top with the beef, cucumber and carrot slaw, edamame, cabbage (if using), and a drizzle of peanut sauce. Garnish with sesame seeds and cilantro and serve immediately with lime wedges and additional peanut sauce on the side.

Yield: 4 servings

Prep Time: 20 minutes, plus 10 minutes to rest falafel

Cook Time: 10 minutes

Falafel Bowls

I first encountered falafel at a small stand outside the gates of Old City Jerusalem, where we ate it piping hot. I was traveling with my family, and my seventeen-year-old self had never tasted a falafel ball before. It was love at first bite, and so began my special love for chickpeas. This is a simple version made with the ever-convenient pantry staple, canned chickpeas. Since it's served bowl-style, I can pack as many veggies as I want into the dish!

FOR THE FALAFEL:

1 (14-ounce) can chickpeas

2 green onions, roughly chopped

1 cup fresh cilantro leaves

½ cup fresh mint leaves

2 cloves garlic, peeled

1 teaspoon kosher salt

1 teaspoon ground cumin

½ teaspoon ground coriander

3 tablespoons all-purpose flour

1 teaspoon baking powder

¼ cup extra-virgin olive oil, plus more if needed, for the pan

FOR THE BOWLS:

4 cups mixed greens

1½ cups chopped cucumbers

1½ cups halved grape tomatoes

½ cup sliced red onions

½ lemon, plus lemon wedges for serving

Extra-virgin olive oil, for drizzling

Kosher salt and freshly ground black pepper

2 pieces pita bread or naan

1 cup tzatziki, homemade (page 76) or store-bought, for serving

1. Rinse and drain the chickpeas and place in a food processor along with the green onions, cilantro, mint, garlic, salt, cumin, and coriander. Pulse until finely chopped but not mushy. Add the flour and baking powder and give it a few more pulses to combine.

2. Using a 2-tablespoon scoop, portion and form the mixture into patties 2 inches in diameter and ½ inch thick, patting them flat with your hand until tightly packed. Let the falafel patties rest for about 10 minutes to give the ingredients time to bind.

3. While the falafel patties rest, toss together the mixed greens, cucumbers, tomatoes, and red onions in a large bowl. Squeeze the lemon half over the salad, then drizzle with olive oil, season to taste with salt and pepper, and toss once more. Set aside.

4. Fry the patties: Heat the olive oil in a skillet, ideally 8 to 10 inches in diameter so that you have about ¼ inch of oil, over medium heat. When the oil is warm, fry the falafel patties in batches until browned on both sides, adding more oil to the pan if needed between batches. Drain the falafel on a paper towel–lined plate.

5. Toast the pita bread or naan and slice into wedges.

6. To serve, place some of the tossed salad in a bowl, top with falafel and pita bread, and serve with tzatziki and lemon wedges.

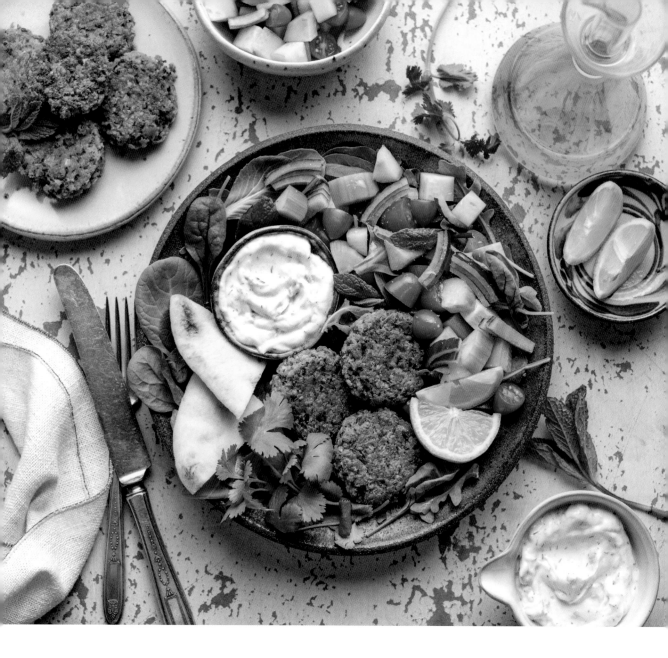

NOTES

Keep the first batch of fried falafel warm in a 175°F oven while you fry the second batch, or until ready to serve.

Cooked falafel can be stored in an airtight container in the refrigerator for up to 5 days. Reheat the falafel in a 175°F oven for 10 minutes.

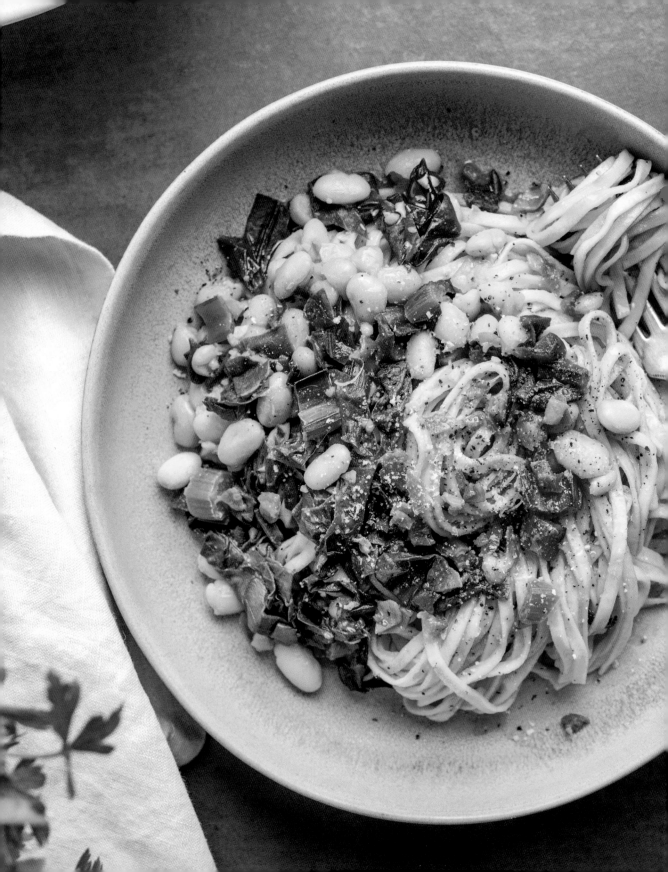

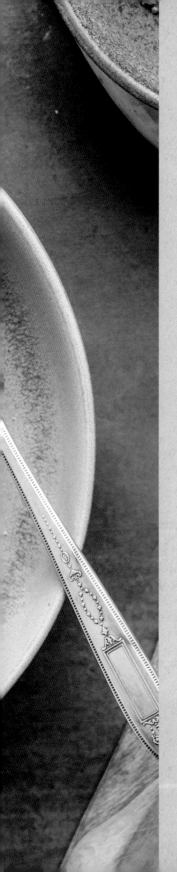

Pasta and Noodles

Stir-Fried Vegetable Chow Mein

Yield: 4 servings
Prep Time: 15 minutes
Cook Time: 20 minutes

Noodles are a must for birthdays and celebrations at our house, but stir-fried noodles is such a simple dish that there's no reason to reserve it for special occasions—it's just as well suited to a weeknight meal! Like most stir-fries, this noodle dish cooks quickly, which is much needed for busy days.

2 tablespoons extra-virgin olive oil, divided

1 cup snow peas

1 cup shredded carrots (about 2 medium carrots)

1 cup diagonally sliced green beans

½ cup diagonally sliced celery

½ cup sliced red bell peppers

½ cup baby corn

1 cup finely chopped yellow onions (about 1 medium onion)

1 tablespoon minced garlic (3 to 4 cloves)

Kosher salt and freshly ground black pepper

2 cups chicken stock

1 cup water

2 tablespoons soy sauce

1 tablespoon Worcestershire sauce

8 ounces chow mein noodles

1 cup thinly sliced napa cabbage

¼ cup fresh cilantro leaves, for garnish

2 tablespoons sliced green onions, for garnish

1 lemon, sliced into wedges, for serving

1. Heat 1 tablespoon of the olive oil in a wok or sauté pan over medium-high heat. Add the snow peas, carrots, green beans, celery, bell peppers, and baby corn and cook for 3 to 4 minutes, stirring frequently, until the vegetables are just tender and still brilliant in color. Transfer the vegetables to a plate and set aside.

2. Lower the heat to medium-low and pour in the remaining tablespoon of olive oil. When the oil is hot, add the onions, garlic, and a pinch each of salt and pepper and cook until the onions are translucent, about 3 minutes.

3. Stir in the chicken stock, water, soy sauce, and Worcestershire sauce and bring to a boil. Lower the heat and let simmer for about 5 minutes.

4. Add the noodles to the wok and cook until soft, 5 to 7 minutes, tossing them as they absorb the sauce. If the noodles are too dry, add a little water. When the noodles are soft, stir in the cabbage and reserved vegetables, tossing to combine. Cook for another minute or so.

5. Transfer the noodles to a serving dish and garnish with the cilantro and green onions. Serve immediately with the lemon wedges.

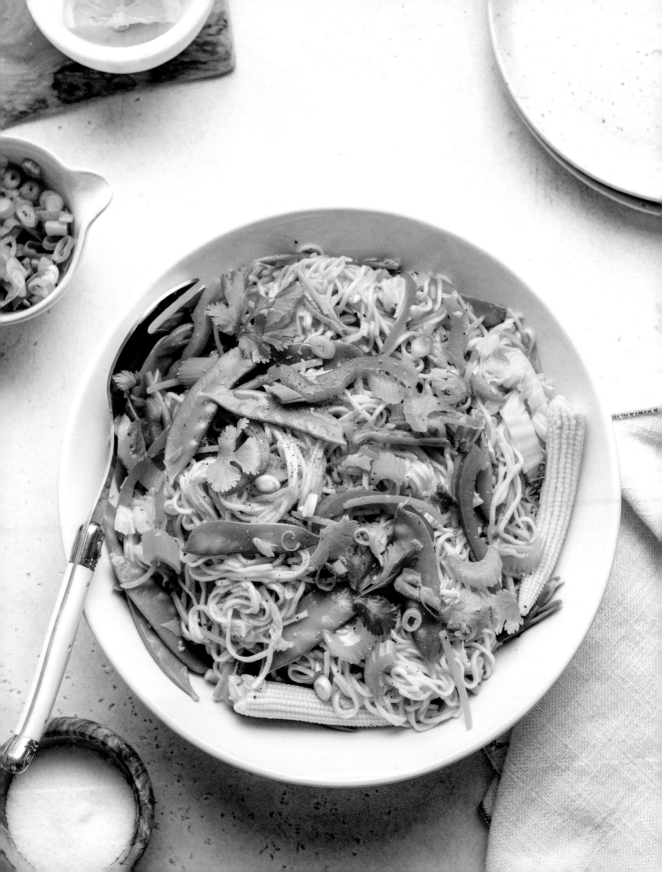

Coconut Zucchini Noodles *with* Shrimp

Yield: 4 servings
Prep Time: 10 minutes
Cook Time: 20 minutes

When zucchini is in season, one of my favorite ways to enjoy it is as zoodles! These days, it's easy to find presliced zucchini noodles in the produce section, making this recipe a cinch to make even if you don't have a spiralizer. The zoodles are cooked in a fragrant coconut broth and served with sautéed shrimp for a deliciously light meal.

FOR THE BROTH AND NOODLES:

1 tablespoon extra-virgin olive oil

1 large shallot, finely chopped (about ½ cup)

1 clove garlic, minced

1 (1-inch) piece fresh ginger, peeled

1 (3-inch) piece lemongrass (from bottom third of stalk)

2 cups chicken stock, heated

1 (13.5-ounce) can light coconut milk

2 tablespoons chopped fresh cilantro, plus more for garnish if desired

1 tablespoon fish sauce

Freshly ground black pepper

3 medium zucchini, spiral-sliced into noodles

FOR THE SHRIMP:

1 tablespoon extra-virgin olive oil

1 pound medium shrimp, peeled and deveined

½ teaspoon fish sauce

Freshly ground black pepper

1. Heat the olive oil in a large saucepan over medium-low heat. Sauté the shallot, garlic, and ginger until the shallot is translucent, about 4 minutes.

2. Place the blade of a chef's knife flat on the lemongrass and pound until the lemongrass is lightly crushed and the stalk is bruised. Stir it into the pan along with the chicken stock and coconut milk. Increase the heat to medium and bring the broth to a simmer; continue to simmer for 10 minutes to give the flavors time to develop.

3. Cook the shrimp: Heat the olive oil in a medium skillet over medium heat. Add the shrimp and cook for 1 minute, then season with the fish sauce and a pinch of pepper. When the shrimp are golden on one side, carefully turn and cook for 1 minute more. Transfer the shrimp to a plate.

4. When the broth has had time to simmer and is fragrant, discard the ginger and lemongrass, stir in the cilantro and fish sauce, and season to taste with pepper. Drop in the zucchini noodles and cook for 3 minutes, or until just tender. Be careful not to overcook the noodles, as they can get mushy. Mix in the shrimp and let them heat through.

5. Serve immediately with an extra sprinkling of cilantro, if desired.

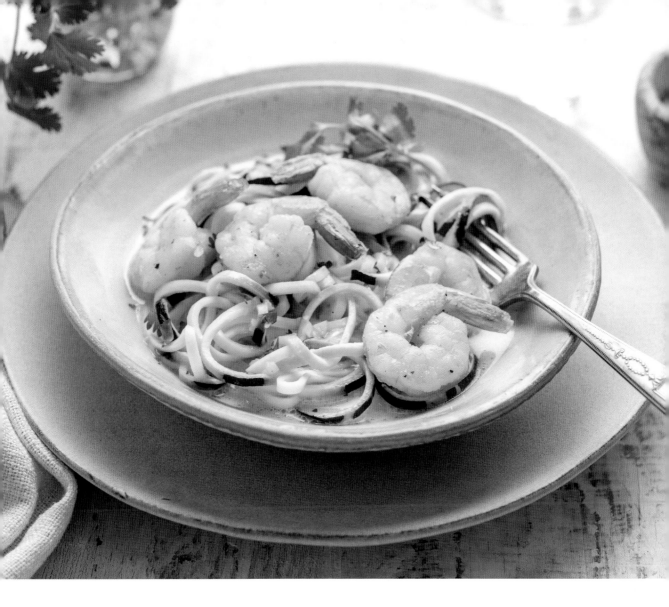

NOTES

When selecting zucchini for spiraling into noodles, choose those that are about 2 inches in diameter. Having a little more surface area in contact with the blades of the spiralizer is helpful when slicing the zucchini into noodles.

Zucchini noodles can be spiralized in advance. After spiraling, pat the zoodles dry with a paper towel, then store in an airtight container in the refrigerator for up to 5 days or in a freezer-safe container in the freezer for up to 12 months.

Brown Butter Orzo *with* **Mushrooms** *and* Kale

Yield: 4 to 6 servings

Prep Time: 10 minutes

Cook Time: 20 minutes

Brown butter is magical. That's all there is to say. My brother harnesses the magic of brown butter in his chocolate chip cookies, but I like to go the savory route. This brown butter orzo is my idea of the perfect dish, with a subtle nuttiness that comes from coaxing butter from its golden hues to toasty darkness.

1 cup orzo

5 tablespoons unsalted butter, sliced

8 ounces cremini mushrooms, sliced

Kosher salt

2 ounces pancetta or bacon, chopped

4 cloves garlic, minced

2½ cups chopped kale

Freshly ground black pepper

2 teaspoons chopped fresh flat-leaf parsley, for garnish

Grated Parmigiano-Reggiano cheese, for garnish (optional)

1. Bring a small pot of salted water to a boil over high heat. Cook the orzo for about 9 minutes, until al dente. Drain and set aside.

2. Melt the butter in a sauté pan over medium heat. Cook until it begins to foam and sizzle and the color deepens to a light to medium brown shade. Keep a close eye on it so it doesn't blacken. Browning the butter should take about 5 minutes.

3. Add the mushrooms, season lightly with salt, and cook until tender.

4. Add the pancetta and garlic and cook until the pancetta is crispy and the garlic is fragrant.

5. Stir in the orzo and kale and season to taste with salt and pepper. Garnish with the parsley and grated Parmigiano-Reggiano cheese, if desired.

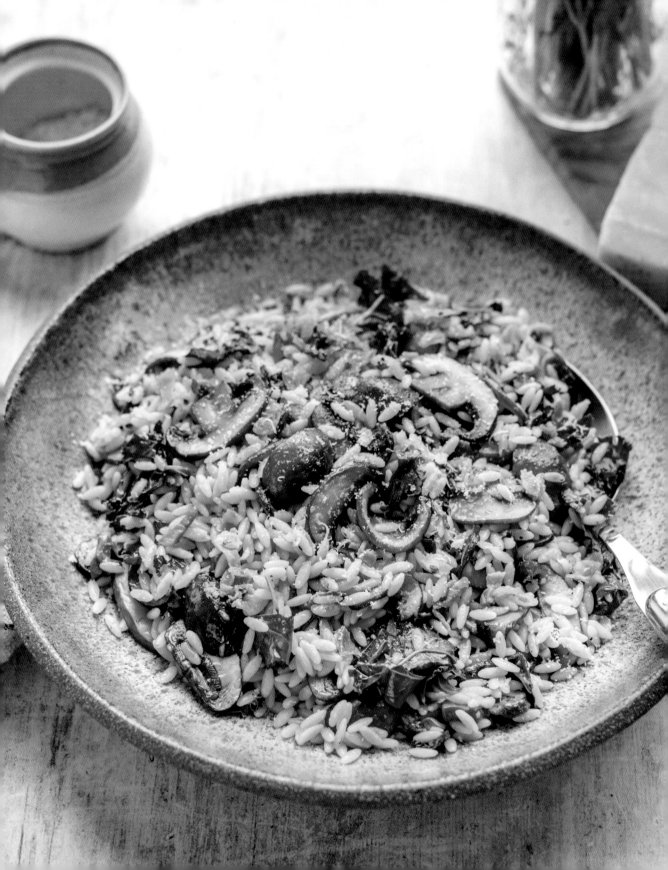

Yield: 6 to 8 servings

Prep Time: 10 minutes

Cook Time: 1 hour

Eggplant Lasagna

When I was a little girl, my mother used to sneak eggplant and mushrooms into her lasagna, knowing that we would gobble it up without thought or protest. These days, I don't bother sneaking around—with ribbons of eggplant serving as the noodles themselves, it can shine front and center! This lasagna is perfect for eggplant lovers...and those who want a low-carb, gluten-free lasagna.

2 large eggplants

3 tablespoons extra-virgin olive oil, divided

Kosher salt and freshly ground black pepper

6 ounces pancetta, chopped

6 ounces kale, chopped

1 (15-ounce) container whole milk ricotta

1 large egg, lightly beaten

1 cup grated Parmigiano-Reggiano cheese, plus more for garnish

1 (28-ounce) jar marinara sauce

1 cup shredded mozzarella cheese (see Notes, page 67)

1 tablespoon finely chopped fresh flat-leaf parsley, for garnish

Prepare the eggplant:

1. Preheat the oven to 400°F with a rack placed in the center of the oven. Line a sheet pan with parchment paper.

2. Using a mandoline or a sharp knife, carefully cut the eggplant lengthwise into slices about ½ inch thick. Brush the slices on both sides with 2½ tablespoons of the olive oil and season generously with salt and pepper. Roast the eggplant, flipping the slices once halfway through, for 20 to 25 minutes, or until tender and pliable. Remove from the oven and lower the oven temperature to 375°F.

Prepare the filling:

3. While the eggplant roasts, heat the remaining ½ tablespoon of oil in a sauté pan over medium heat. Cook the pancetta until browned and crispy, stirring periodically. Drain the excess fat, leaving about 1 teaspoon in the pan with the pancetta.

4. Add the kale, season with a pinch of pepper, and cook until wilted. Transfer the pancetta and kale to a medium bowl. Stir in the ricotta, egg, and Parmigiano-Reggiano cheese and season with a pinch of pepper.

Assemble the lasagna:

5. Pour 1 cup of the marinara sauce into a 9 by 13 by 3¼-inch (or 4-quart) baking dish. Place a layer of eggplant on top, then spread on half of the ricotta mixture. Sprinkle with one-third of the mozzarella cheese, followed by another layer of marinara sauce. Repeat the layers, finishing with mozzarella.

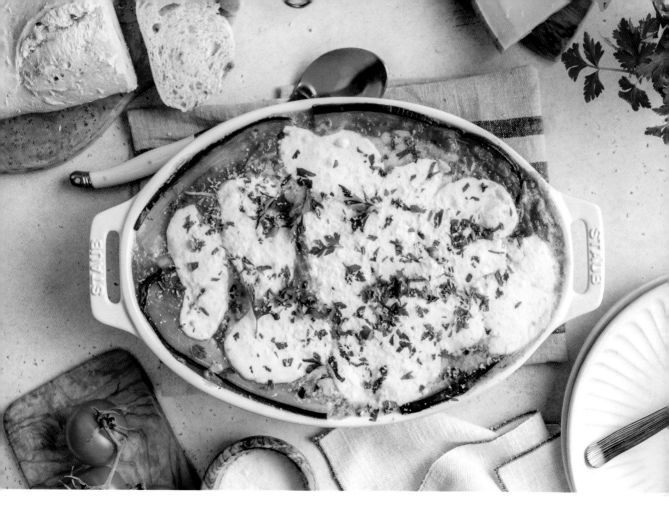

6. Bake for 30 to 35 minutes, or until the top is golden and the sauce is bubbling. Remove from the oven and let sit for 10 minutes. Garnish with more Parmigiano-Reggiano cheese and the parsley. Serve immediately.

NOTES

Eggplant can release a lot of water. If you find that your eggplant has done so after roasting, pat it dry with paper towels before assembling the lasagna. For this reason, it is best to assemble the lasagna right before baking.

You can prepare the eggplant and filling components up to a day in advance and store them separately in the refrigerator until you are ready to assemble and bake the lasagna.

Linguine *with* Beans *and* Swiss Chard

Yield: 4 servings

Prep Time: 10 minutes

Cook Time: 20 minutes

Sometimes you just need to make a pantry-friendly meal—I always make sure to have canned beans on hand for nourishing recipes like this one! Swiss chard is so simple to sauté and is packed with vitamins, adding wonderful nutrients to this humble pasta dish.

9 ounces linguine

Kosher salt

2 large bunches Swiss chard

1 tablespoon extra-virgin olive oil

1 ounce prosciutto, chopped

3 cloves garlic, minced

Freshly ground black pepper

1 (15-ounce) can cannellini beans, drained and rinsed

2 to 8 tablespoons chicken stock

¼ cup grated Parmigiano-Reggiano cheese

1. Bring a large pot of water to a boil over high heat. Season generously with salt. Cook the linguine until al dente, following the package directions. Drain and set aside.

2. While the pasta cooks, rinse the Swiss chard thoroughly. Cut or tear the leaves away from the stalks and give the leaves a rough chop.

3. Heat the olive oil in a sauté pan over medium heat. When the oil is shimmering, add the prosciutto and cook until crispy. Remove the prosciutto from the pan and set aside.

4. Add the garlic to the pan and cook until golden brown and fragrant, about 1 minute. Stir in the Swiss chard and season with a pinch each of salt and pepper. Cook the Swiss chard, stirring periodically, until it begins to wilt, 3 to 4 minutes.

5. Add the cooked pasta, beans, and 2 tablespoons of chicken stock and season to taste with salt and pepper. If the pasta seems too dry, add up to 6 tablespoons more stock as necessary, 1 tablespoon at a time.

6. Transfer the pasta to a serving bowl, sprinkle with the cheese, and enjoy.

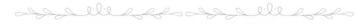

NOTE

Any white bean works well in this recipe. I love using cannellini beans, but you can also use Great Northern beans, navy beans, or your favorite white beans.

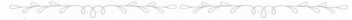

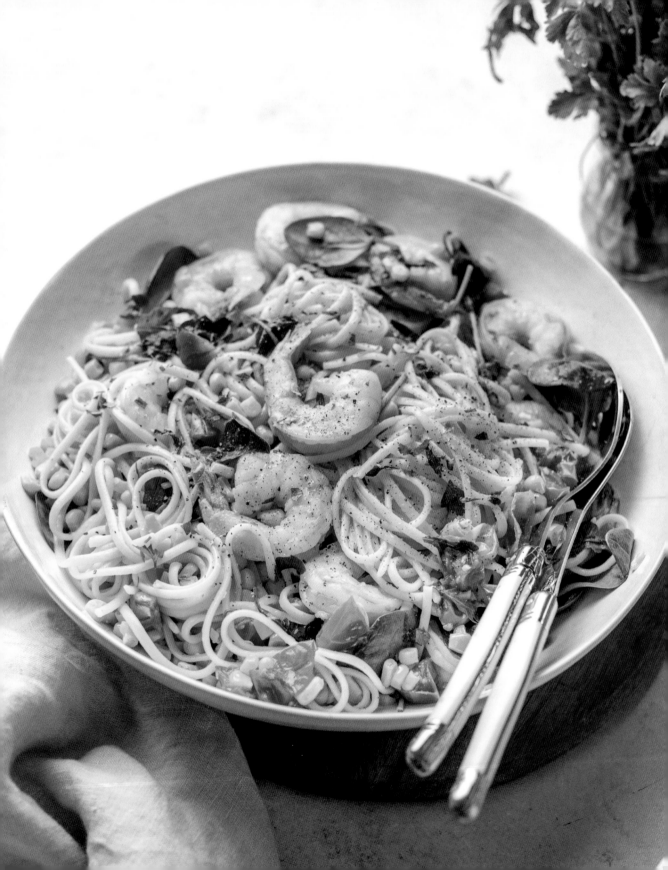

Garlicky Sweet Potato Noodles *with* Vegetable Ragu

Yield: 4 servings

Prep Time: 15 minutes

Cook Time: 30 minutes

If you've never had sweet potato noodles, you're in for a treat. I find spiralized sweet potatoes extremely satisfying—they fill you up like pasta but are so much better for you! And while this vegetable ragu would be equally tasty with pasta, it is utterly delicious with sweet potato noodles.

4 tablespoons extra-virgin olive oil, divided

½ cup diced yellow onions (about ½ medium onion)

½ cup diced carrots

½ cup diced celery

6 cloves garlic, minced, divided

1 tablespoon tomato paste

2 teaspoons balsamic vinegar

¼ cup chopped mushrooms

¼ cup diced eggplant

¼ cup diced red bell peppers

¼ cup diced yellow squash

¼ cup diced zucchini

¼ cup red lentils

1 cup canned crushed tomatoes

¾ cup plus 2 to 4 tablespoons chicken or vegetable stock, divided

2 medium sweet potatoes, spiralized

½ teaspoon kosher salt

Grated or shaved Parmigiano-Reggiano cheese, for garnish

Fresh basil leaves, for garnish

1. Heat 2 tablespoons of the olive oil in a large saucepan over medium heat. Add the onions, carrots, celery, and half of the minced garlic. Cook until the onions have softened, about 5 minutes.

2. Stir in the tomato paste, vinegar, vegetables, lentils, crushed tomatoes, and ¾ cup of the stock. Bring to a boil, then lower the heat to a simmer and cook until the vegetables and lentils are tender, about 20 minutes.

3. In a deep-sided skillet or sauté pan, gently cook the remaining garlic in the remaining 2 tablespoons of olive oil over medium-low heat. Be careful not to burn the garlic.

4. When the garlic is golden brown, drop in the sweet potato noodles, tossing to coat in the garlicky oil, and season with the salt. Cook for 2 minutes, or until tender, gently stirring periodically.

5. Add 2 tablespoons of the stock to the skillet, cover, and cook for another 2 minutes to soften the noodles. If the pan becomes dry before the noodles have softened, add the remaining stock, 1 tablespoon at a time; just be careful because the noodles can go from crispy to mushy very quickly.

6. Serve the sweet potato noodles with the vegetable ragu and garnish with Parmigiano-Reggiano cheese and basil leaves.

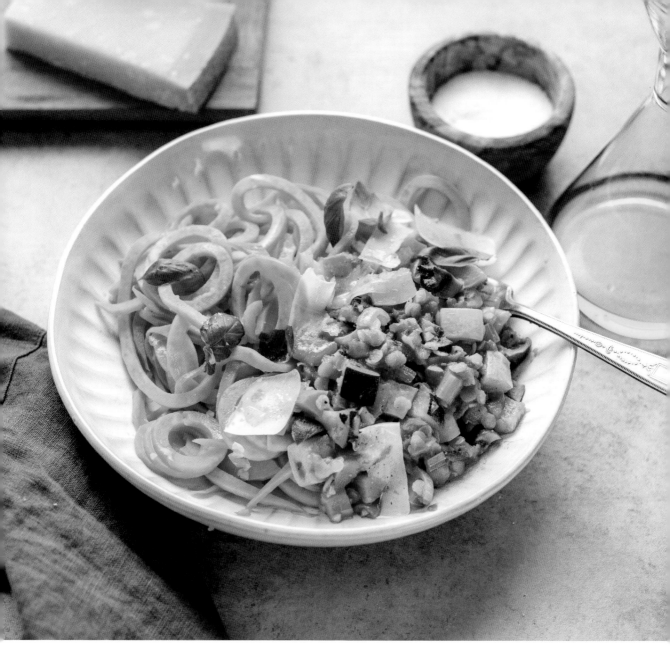

NOTE

The vegetable ragu can be made a few days in advance. Store the cooled ragu in a tightly sealed container in the refrigerator. With the ragu prepped, the dish comes together even faster, since the sweet potato noodles take just a few minutes to cook.

Somen Noodles in a Creamy Coconut Broth *with* Bok Choy

Yield: 2 servings
Prep Time: 20 minutes
Cook Time: 20 minutes

When you have a well-stocked pantry, a cozy meal is never far away, and this dish is a prime example. I always keep dried shiitake mushrooms on hand, which, once rehydrated, have far more flavor than fresh ones. Somen noodles, chicken stock, and coconut milk are also pantry basics. All that's needed to round out the dish are some vibrant greens. Bok choy is perfect in this deliciously fragrant noodle soup, but feel free to drop in whatever greens you have!

1 ounce dried shiitake mushrooms

2 bundles somen noodles (about 7 ounces)

1 tablespoon extra-virgin olive oil

10 ounces bok choy, chopped, stems and leaves divided

1 large shallot, finely chopped (about ½ cup)

1 clove garlic, minced

1 (1-inch) piece fresh ginger, peeled

1 (3-inch) piece lemongrass (from bottom third of stalk), pounded with the flat of the blade of a chef's knife

2½ cups chicken or seafood stock, heated

1 (13.5-ounce) can light coconut milk

2 tablespoons chopped fresh cilantro

1 tablespoon fish sauce

Freshly ground black pepper

Red chili pepper, thinly sliced, for garnish (optional)

1. Place the dried shiitakes in a bowl and cover with boiling water. Let soak until they are plump and rehydrated, about 20 minutes. Drain the water. Cut off and discard the stems and slice the mushroom caps into strips.

2. Bring a large pot of water to a rolling boil. Drop in the somen noodles and cook according to the package directions, about 3 minutes. Drain the noodles, rinse well under cold water, and divide the noodles between two serving bowls.

3. Heat the olive oil in a large saucepan over low heat. Cook the bok choy stems with the shallot, garlic, ginger, and lemongrass until the shallot has wilted and the aromatics are fragrant. Stir in the stock, coconut milk, and bok choy leaves. Bring to a simmer and cook for 10 minutes. Discard the ginger and lemongrass, then stir in the cilantro and fish sauce and season with black pepper to taste.

4. Ladle the hot broth and bok choy over the noodles. Garnish with red chili slices, if desired, and serve.

NOTE

When storing leftovers, place the broth and noodles in separate containers; otherwise, the noodles will absorb all the broth. To reheat the noodles, pour boiling water over them to loosen them, then drain and serve with the broth and toppings.

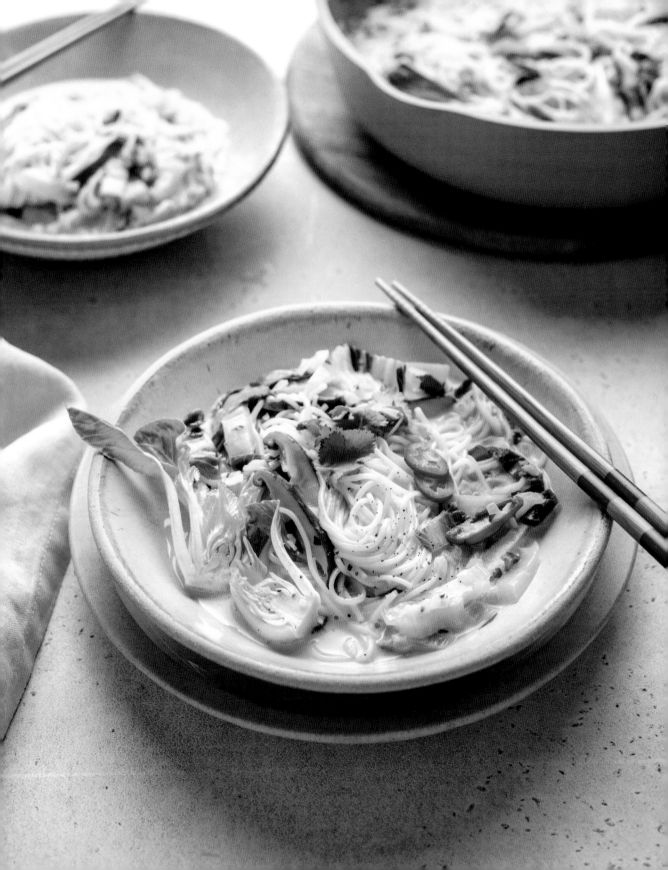

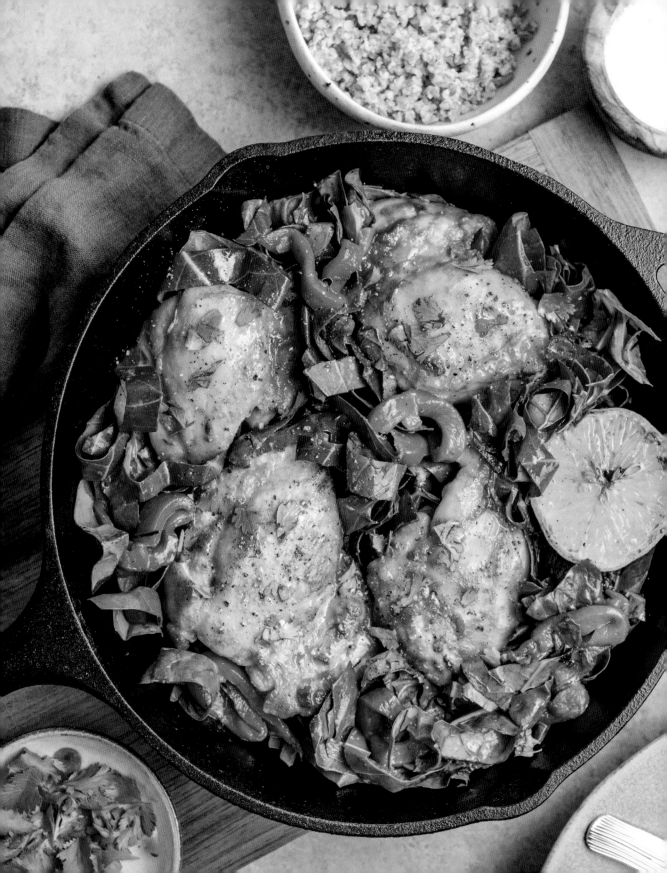

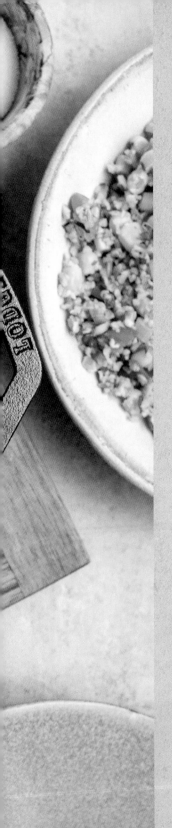

Hearty Plates

Broccoli Rice Chicken Skillet

Yield: 4 servings

Prep Time: 5 minutes

Cook Time: 35 minutes

Cauliflower rice gets all the glory, but if you were to ask my kids, broccoli rice is so much better! Granted, they're a bit partial to broccoli, but I have to agree; it's a beautifully green and nutritious alternative to plain old rice. This chicken skillet is finished off in the oven, giving the broccoli rice time to toast up for a little extra texture.

1 teaspoon kosher salt

1 teaspoon smoked paprika

½ teaspoon ground coriander

½ teaspoon ground cumin

3 boneless chicken thighs, preferably skin-on (about 14 ounces)

1 large head broccoli

3 tablespoons extra-virgin olive oil, divided

1 tablespoon unsalted butter

¼ cup finely diced yellow onions

2 cloves garlic, minced

3 tablespoons chicken stock

1 cup grated Parmigiano-Reggiano cheese

Freshly ground black pepper

Chopped fresh flat-leaf parsley, for garnish (optional)

Lemon slices, for garnish (optional)

1. Preheat the oven to 450°F with a rack placed in the center of the oven.

2. In a small bowl, mix together the salt, paprika, coriander, and cumin. Rub the spice mixture liberally all over the chicken and set aside.

3. Trim and discard the leaves and tough base of the broccoli stalk. Cut off the florets and set aside. Peel and discard the skin of the broccoli stalk and roughly chop the stalk into 1-inch chunks.

4. Place the broccoli stalks in a food processor. Pulse until chopped, then add the florets and continue to pulse until the broccoli has a texture reminiscent of rice. Set aside.

5. Heat 2 tablespoons of the olive oil in a large cast-iron skillet or other heavy ovenproof pan over high heat until hot but not smoking. Add the chicken; if using skin-on thighs, place them skin side down. Sear for 3 to 4 minutes, then lower the heat to medium-high. Flip the chicken over, cook for about 2 minutes, then transfer the pan to the oven and roast for 15 minutes, or until the chicken reaches an internal temperature of 165°F.

6. While the chicken roasts, heat the remaining tablespoon of olive oil and the butter in a separate skillet. Add the onions and garlic and season with a pinch of salt. Cook until the onions are translucent, about 5 minutes. Stir in the broccoli rice, chicken stock, and cheese and season to taste with salt and pepper.

7. When the chicken is about 5 minutes from being fully cooked, nestle the broccoli rice in the skillet around the chicken and return it to the oven to finish cooking. Slice the roasted chicken into strips before serving. Garnish with parsley and lemon slices, if desired.

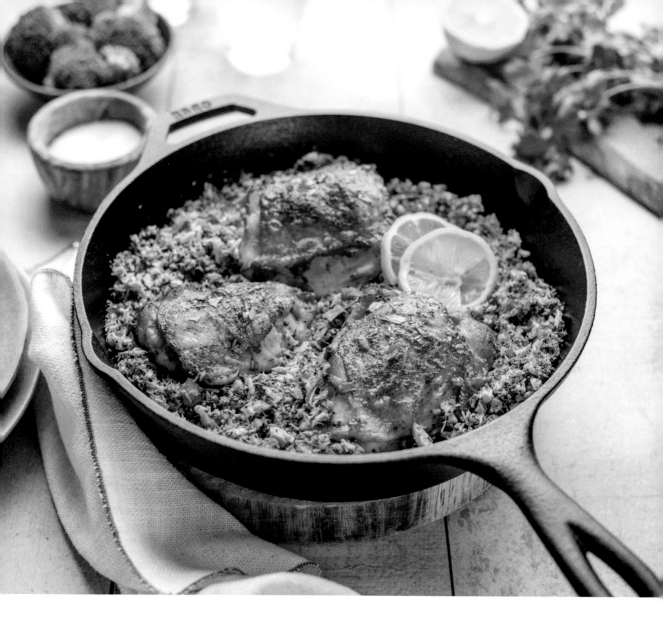

NOTES

The broccoli rice can be prepped ahead of time and stored in an airtight container in the refrigerator for up to 3 days.

Boneless, skinless chicken thighs are commonly found in the meat department, but it seems a shame since there's so much flavor in the skin. If you wish to use boneless chicken thighs with the skin on, I recommend stopping by the butcher counter and asking the butcher to debone some skin-on thighs for you.

Turkey Tater Tot Casserole

Yield: 4 to 6 servings
Prep Time: 5 minutes
Cook Time: 1 hour

I fell in love with tater tot casserole as a grad student in the Midwest. My friends Robin, Liz, Beth, and I would take turns hosting dinner every Thursday, and we'd happily study and eat together, usually comfort foods that reminded us of home. When we went to Robin's place, we always begged her to make her tater tot casserole. This is my take on it, swapping out beef for lean ground turkey and adding a medley of mixed vegetables. It's instant comfort!

2½ tablespoons extra-virgin olive oil, divided

1 cup finely chopped yellow onions (about 1 medium onion)

Kosher salt

8 ounces mushrooms, chopped

3 teaspoons soy sauce, divided

8 ounces ground turkey breast

Freshly ground black pepper

¼ cup (½ stick) unsalted butter

¼ cup all-purpose flour

2 cups vegetable stock

½ cup whole milk or almond milk (unsweetened and unflavored)

4 cups frozen mixed vegetables

1 (16-ounce) package frozen tater tots

Chopped fresh flat-leaf parsley, for garnish

1. Preheat the oven to 425°F with a rack placed in the center of the oven.

2. Heat 1½ tablespoons of the olive oil in a heavy skillet over medium-low heat, then add the onions and season with a pinch of salt. Cook until translucent, about 5 minutes. Increase the heat to medium-high, add the mushrooms, and sauté for about 2 minutes. Add 2 teaspoons of the soy sauce and continue to sauté until the mushroom liquid has evaporated. Remove the mushrooms from the pan and set aside.

3. Heat the remaining tablespoon of oil in the same skillet over medium heat. Add the turkey and season with the remaining teaspoon of soy sauce and a generous pinch of pepper. Cook, breaking up the meat into crumbles, until the turkey is fully cooked and no longer pink, about 5 minutes, then add it to the cooked mushrooms.

4. Melt the butter in a medium saucepan over low heat and sprinkle the flour on top. When the flour starts to bubble, whisk continuously to create a roux, about 2 minutes. Add the vegetable stock while whisking, increase the heat to high, and bring to a boil. Continue to whisk until the sauce is free of lumps. Add the milk and whisk to combine; simmer over medium-low heat, until the sauce has thickened, about 5 minutes.

5. Add the reserved mushroom and turkey mixture and the frozen mixed vegetables. Adjust the seasoning with salt and pepper to taste.

6. Transfer the mixture to a shallow 1-quart baking dish (a 9-inch round tart pan is ideal). Arrange the tater tots in a single layer on top and lightly cover with foil. Bake for

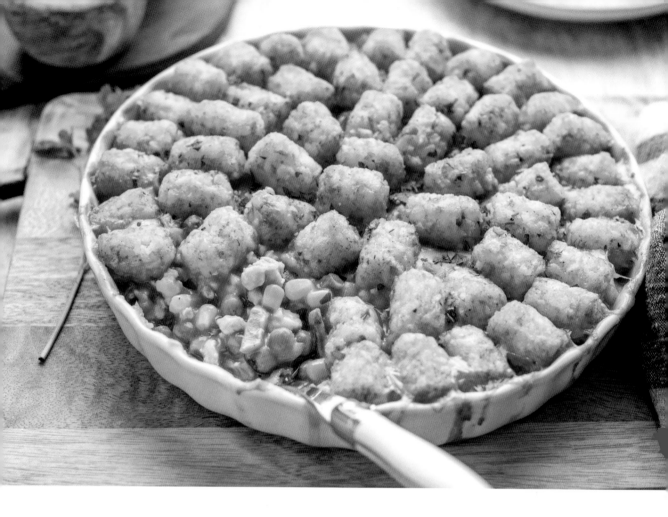

about 30 minutes. Remove the foil and bake for another 10 minutes, or until the filling is bubbling and the tater tots are golden brown.

7. Serve immediately, garnished with parsley.

NOTES

Tater tots are a generic household name, but because the name is a registered trademark, you may find it in your freezer section labeled as "potato tots," "potato puffs," or "spud puppies," depending on where you are located.

For this casserole, I opt for a shallow baking dish to allow the tater tots to brown beautifully on all sides. If you don't have a tart pan or similar, you can use a 9-inch pie pan or a 9- or 10-inch ovenproof skillet.

Spinach Risotto with Scallops

There was a time when the idea of making risotto seemed daunting to me—so many recipes out there come with warnings about continual stirring, leaving us to assume that risotto is horribly fussy. Let me assure you that it's not. And if you have a pressure cooker, making the perfect risotto is even easier! I like to infuse my risotto with healthy spinach, turning it a beautiful shade of green, and serve it topped with juicy seared scallops. It's an elegant meal that really is easier than you think.

FOR THE RISOTTO:

2 tablespoons extra-virgin olive oil

1½ cups finely chopped yellow onions

2 cloves garlic, minced

1½ cups short-grain rice, such as Arborio

5 cups chicken stock, divided

8 cups packed baby spinach

1 tablespoon chopped fresh flat-leaf parsley

1 teaspoon fresh thyme leaves

½ cup grated Parmigiano-Reggiano cheese

1 tablespoon unsalted butter

Kosher salt and freshly ground black pepper

FOR THE SCALLOPS:

2 teaspoons extra-virgin olive oil

1 pound sea scallops

Kosher salt and freshly ground black pepper

1. *Make the risotto:*

   STOVETOP METHOD: Heat the olive oil in a medium saucepan over medium-low heat. Add the onions and garlic and cook until the onions are translucent, about 5 minutes. Stir in the rice and toast for a minute or so, stirring to make sure the grains are coated. Stir in 2 cups of the chicken stock and cook until the liquid is nearly absorbed, stirring frequently. Set aside ½ cup of the stock for the spinach puree, then continue adding the remaining stock, about 1 cup at a time, when the liquid is nearly absorbed, stirring often. This process should take about 25 minutes; the rice will be tender and creamy.

   PRESSURE COOKER METHOD: Heat the olive oil in a pressure cooker set to the sauté function. Add the onions and garlic and cook until the onions are translucent, about 5 minutes. Stir in the rice and toast for a minute or so, stirring to make sure the grains are coated. Stir in 4½ cups of the chicken stock. Cover with the valve set to pressure and cook on the risotto setting for 6 minutes. Depressurize the pressure cooker, then remove the lid. If the risotto seems a touch watery, simply simmer the risotto, uncovered, on the sauté function for about 5 minutes, until it has thickened to your desired consistency.

   Make the spinach puree and finish the risotto:

2. Bring the remaining ½ cup of stock to a simmer in a medium saucepan over medium heat. Add the spinach in batches, letting it wilt down before adding more. Transfer to a food processor and pulse until smooth.

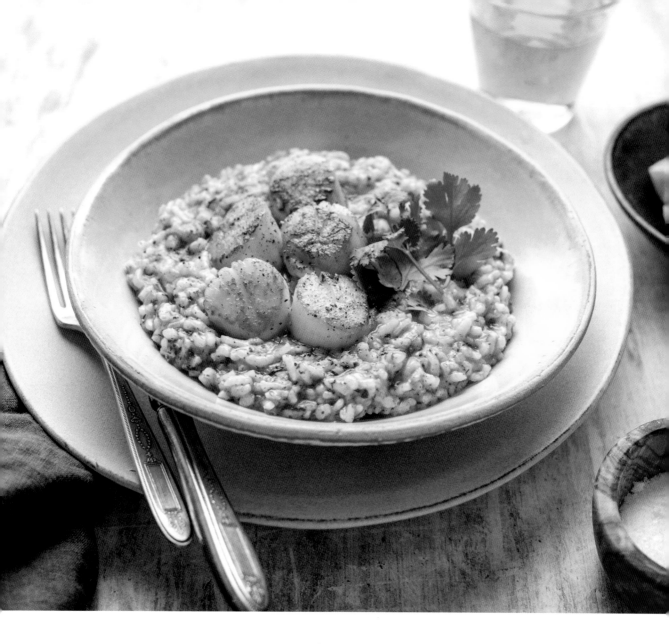

3. Stir the spinach puree, parsley, thyme, cheese, and butter into the risotto. Season to taste with salt and pepper.

Sear the scallops:

4. Heat a large nonstick skillet over medium-high heat, then pour in the olive oil. Lightly season the scallops with salt and pepper. Working in batches, sear the scallops for about 2 minutes, until golden brown on one side. Flip and cook until golden brown on the other side, 2 to 3 minutes more. Serve on top of the spinach risotto.

Winter Vegetable Shepherd's Pie

Yield: 6 servings
Prep Time: 20 minutes
Cook Time: 50 minutes

Shepherd's pie may have started out as a frugal dish loaded with hearty ground meat and blanketed in a mashed potato crust, but I think that once you try this version, which flip-flops the ratio of meat to vegetables, you'll agree that it's worth altering the classic at least once in a while. I throw in all the winter vegetables I can find, giving parsnips, sweet potatoes, and Brussels sprouts a chance to shine.

FOR THE FILLING:

1 tablespoon extra-virgin olive oil, plus more for the baking dish

1 cup minced yellow onions (about 1 medium onion)

2 cloves garlic, minced

8 ounces 85% lean ground beef

2 teaspoons kosher salt

2 teaspoons Worcestershire sauce

1 teaspoon balsamic vinegar

1 cup trimmed and quartered Brussels sprouts

1 cup diced carrots (about 2 medium carrots)

1 cup diced celery (about 2 medium stalks)

1 cup chopped mushrooms

1 cup diced parsnips

1 cup diced sweet potatoes

2 tablespoons all-purpose flour

1 tablespoon tomato paste

1 cup beef stock

1 bay leaf

Sprig of fresh thyme

Dash of Tabasco sauce

Kosher salt and freshly ground black pepper

FOR THE MASHED POTATO TOPPING:

1½ pounds russet potatoes (about 4 potatoes), peeled and quartered lengthwise

¼ cup (½ stick) unsalted butter

⅓ cup whole milk, plus more if needed

Kosher salt and freshly ground black pepper

1 tablespoon chopped fresh flat-leaf parsley, for garnish

1. Preheat the oven to 400°F with a rack placed in the center of the oven. Lightly grease a 1-quart baking dish with olive oil.

Make the filling:

2. Heat the olive oil in a sauté pan over medium heat. Add the onions and garlic and cook, stirring frequently, until the onions have softened, about 5 minutes. Add the ground beef and cook, breaking it up into crumbles and stirring frequently, until browned.

3. Stir in the salt, Worcestershire sauce, and vinegar, followed by the vegetables. Cook until the mushrooms have softened, about 5 minutes.

4. Stir in the flour and cook for about 1 minute.

5. Add the tomato paste, beef stock, bay leaf, thyme, and Tabasco. Bring to a boil, then lower the heat to a simmer. Cover the pan and simmer for 10 to 15 minutes, until

(recipe continues on page 195)

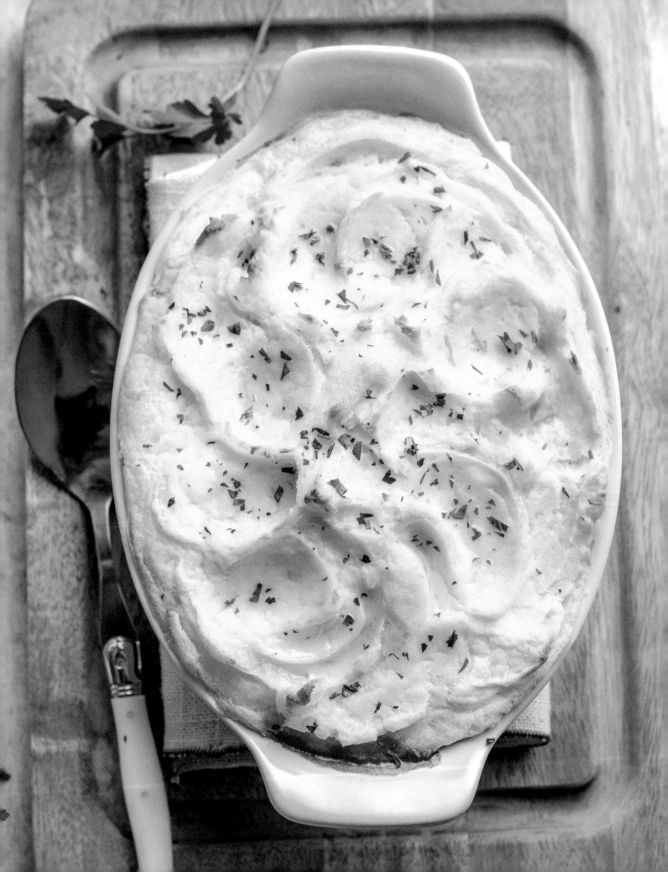

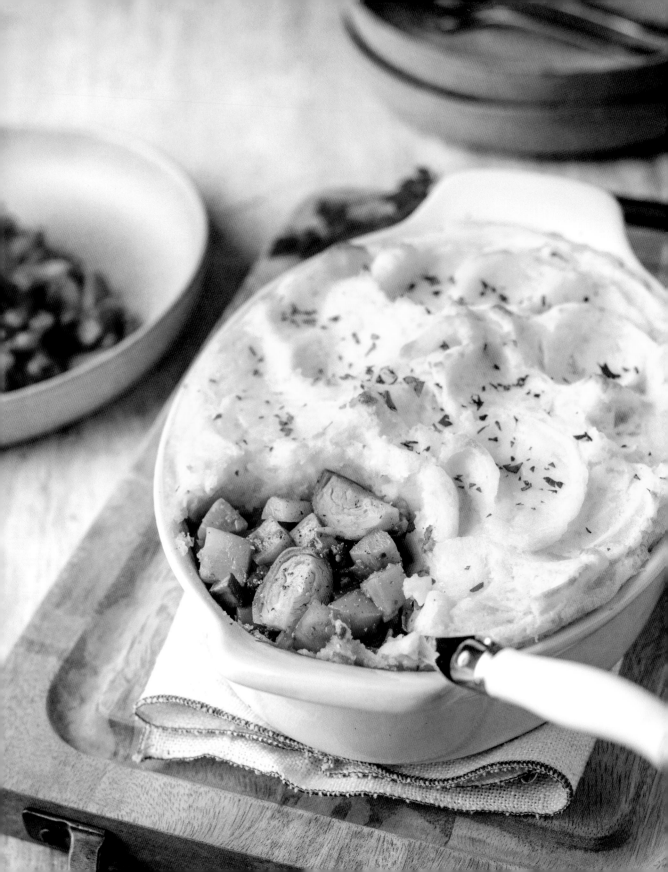

the sauce has thickened slightly. Discard the bay leaf and thyme sprig and season the filling to taste with salt and pepper.

Meanwhile, make the potato topping:

Place the quartered potatoes in a large saucepan and pour in enough water to cover the potatoes by about 1 inch. Bring to a boil and cook until the potatoes are fork-tender, 10 to 15 minutes. Drain the potatoes and return them to the saucepan over medium heat. Give any remaining water in the saucepan a chance to evaporate, about 1 minute, then turn off the heat. Add the butter and milk and mash the potatoes to your desired consistency. If the potatoes need a little more moisture, mash in a touch more milk. Season with salt and pepper to taste and set aside.

Assemble:

6. Transfer the filling to the prepared baking dish. Spread the mashed potatoes on top and bake for 25 minutes, until the potato topping has browned and the filling is bubbling. Remove from the oven and let rest for 10 minutes before serving. Sprinkle the parsley on top and enjoy.

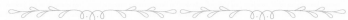

NOTE

If you have leftover mashed potatoes, this is a perfect way to use them—and it makes prep even easier!

Jambalaya Skillet

Yield: 6 servings
Prep Time: 15 minutes
Cook Time: 50 minutes

When I think of jambalaya, I think of how I can truly appreciate the rich and varied food culture in Louisiana, with its melting pot of flavors, given how my own heritage has been influenced by so many diverse groups. This jambalaya has a few extra ingredients that make it a little more legume and root vegetable heavy, but it still has all the main stars you expect to find in the Creole classic.

3 tablespoons extra-virgin olive oil

1 medium yellow onion, chopped

1 green bell pepper, chopped

1 cup chopped celery (2 to 3 medium stalks)

3 cloves garlic, minced

6 ounces boneless, skinless chicken breasts, cut into 1-inch cubes

Kosher salt and freshly ground black pepper

1 (14-ounce) can pinto beans, drained and rinsed

6 ounces vegan andouille sausage, sliced

½ cup diced sweet potatoes

1 teaspoon Cajun spice blend

1 teaspoon dried thyme leaves, crushed

¼ teaspoon cayenne pepper

1 bay leaf

2 teaspoons chopped fresh flat-leaf parsley, plus more for garnish

1½ cups converted rice

2 cups chicken stock

1 cup tomato sauce

8 ounces small shrimp, peeled and deveined

1. Heat the olive oil in a large skillet over medium heat. Add the onion, bell pepper, celery, and garlic and cook, stirring frequently, until the onion has wilted, about 5 minutes.

2. Add the chicken, season lightly with salt and pepper, and cook for another 5 minutes, until the chicken is nearly cooked. Add the beans, sausage, sweet potatoes, Cajun spice, thyme, cayenne pepper, bay leaf, and parsley and season lightly with salt and pepper. Cook for 1 minute.

3. Stir in the rice, chicken stock, and tomato sauce and bring to a boil. Reduce the heat to medium-low, cover, and cook until the rice is fully cooked, about 30 minutes.

4. Gently stir in the shrimp and cook for about 5 minutes more, until the shrimp are pink and opaque. Adjust the seasoning with salt and pepper to taste.

5. When ready to serve, fluff the rice with a fork. Garnish each serving with additional chopped parsley.

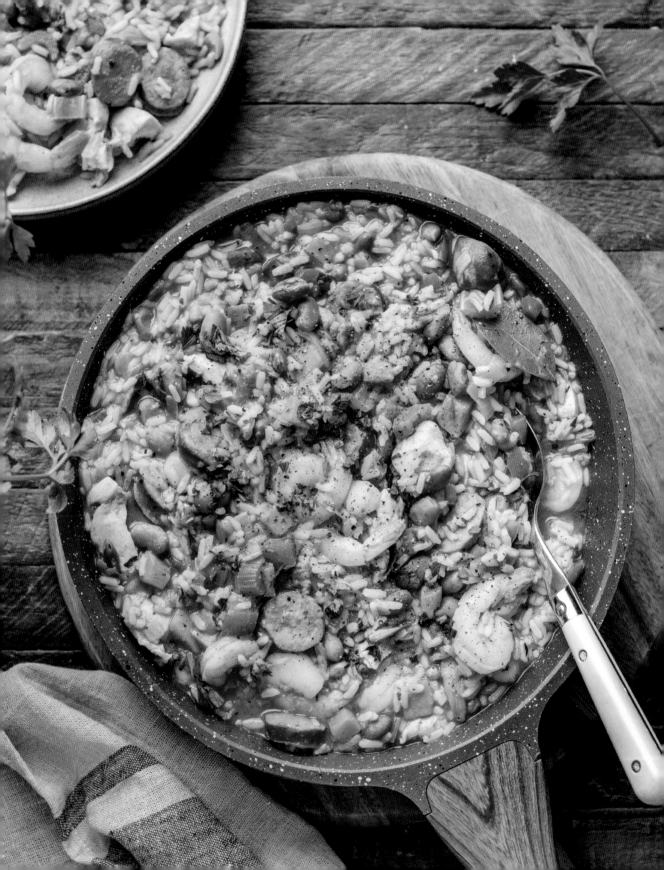

Filipino Pinakbet (Vegetable Pork Stew)

Yield: 4 to 6 servings
Prep Time: 15 minutes
Cook Time: 35 minutes

Pinakbet, a simple Filipino stew that is traditionally vegetable-forward, is usually made with kalabasa (pumpkin), long beans, okra, bitter melon, pork, and sometimes shrimp in a simple broth flavored with shrimp paste. The vegetables are what really shine in this dish, with the proteins playing second fiddle; if you prefer, you can omit the proteins altogether. The beauty of pinakbet is that you can use whatever ingredients are available to you—perfect for cleaning out the vegetable bin! In this version, I replace the pumpkin with kabocha squash and omit the bitter melon to suit my family's preferences, but I make up for it by adding a variety of summer squash.

1½ tablespoons extra-virgin olive oil

½ cup diced yellow onions (about ½ medium onion)

2 cloves garlic, minced

1 (1-inch) piece fresh ginger, peeled

2 medium tomatoes, quartered

8 ounces pork tenderloin, cut into 2-inch cubes

¼ cup shrimp paste or fish sauce, divided (see Notes)

Freshly ground black pepper

2 cups water

½ kabocha squash, peeled, seeded, and cut into 1-inch cubes

3 ounces long beans or string beans, cut into 3-inch pieces

1 cup sliced fresh okra

1 Chinese or Japanese eggplant, cut into ½-inch rounds

1 yellow squash, cut in half lengthwise, then into ½-inch half-moons

1 zucchini, cut in half lengthwise, then into ½-inch half-moons

Kosher salt (if needed)

Cooked white or brown jasmine rice, for serving

1. Heat the olive oil in a small Dutch oven over low heat. Add the onions, garlic, and ginger and cook until the onions are translucent, about 7 minutes.

2. Increase the heat to medium and stir in the tomatoes and pork along with 1 teaspoon of the shrimp paste and pepper to taste. Cook until the tomatoes begin to break down, about 4 minutes.

3. Stir together the remaining shrimp paste and the water and add to the pot along with the kabocha squash. Bring to a boil, then lower the heat to a simmer, cover, and cook until the squash is just tender, about 10 minutes.

4. Add the beans, okra, and eggplant and cook until the eggplant is just tender, about 8 minutes.

(recipe continues on page 201)

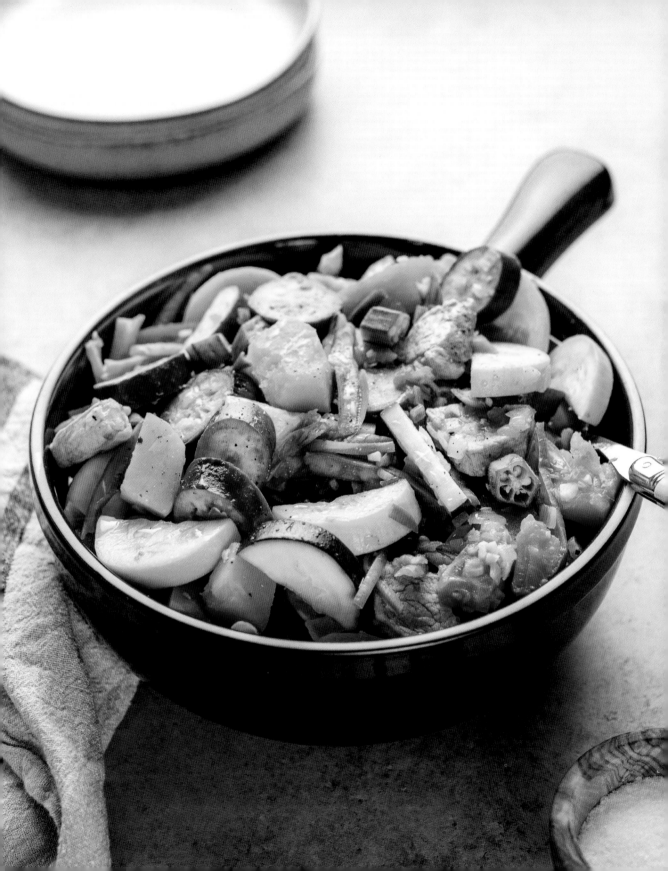

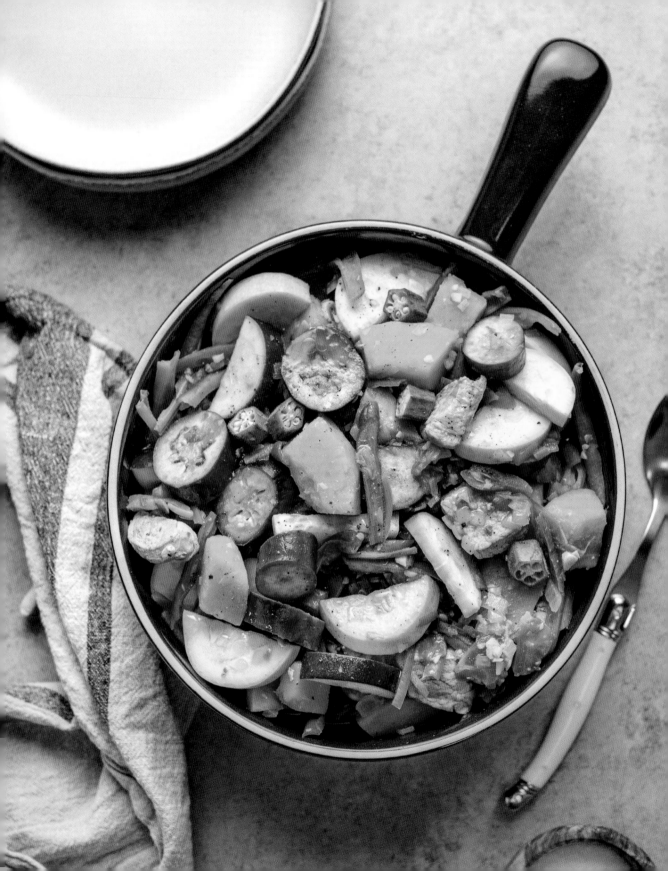

5. Stir in the yellow squash and zucchini and simmer until the squash is fork-tender, about 4 minutes. Adjust the seasoning with salt and pepper to taste if necessary.

6. Serve hot with rice.

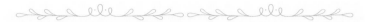

NOTES

The word *pinakbet* originates from the Ilocano word *pinakebbet,* which means "shrunk" or "shriveled," and speaks to how the vegetables shrink as they slowly cook in the simmering broth. The dish can be found beyond the northern Ilocos region of the Philippines and is a quintessential Filipino vegetable dish that can be served as a main dish or a side to your meal.

Fish sauce versus shrimp paste: which should you use?

Shrimp paste, a fermented condiment known as bagoong, is traditional in Filipino pinakbet (and many other dishes). It adds an extra punch of flavor (and umami) to food. You can find it in Asian markets.

Fish sauce is a convenient and excellent substitute for shrimp paste. I always have some in the pantry and often use it as salt—in this dish, it adds extra umami flavor to the simple broth. Since it's readily available in most grocery stores, this is the easier option.

In either case, a little goes a long way in adding delicious flavor. To those who are new to either product, do not be afraid of the pungent smell; I promise it is delicious. I think of both as being similar to anchovies. If you are unable to locate either one, simply season your broth with kosher salt to taste.

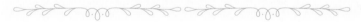

Yield: 4 servings

Prep Time: 15 minutes

Cook Time: 45 minutes

Vegetable Cassoulet

When the temperatures dip, one of my favorite things to make is a cassoulet. Traditionally, cassoulet is a dish that simmers all day long, with dried beans, a hunk of pork shoulder, and morsels of sausage—true comfort food. This is a lightened-up version, and since it's made with significantly less meat and canned beans, it can be made in a fraction of the time. To make the cassoulet even more vegetable-forward, feel free to omit the sausage. It will still have lots of flavor from the bacon and will be just as delicious!

2½ ounces bacon, finely diced

1 cup panko breadcrumbs

1 tablespoon extra-virgin olive oil, plus more for drizzling if desired

1 cup diced carrots (about 2 medium carrots)

1 cup diced celery (about 2 medium stalks)

⅔ cup chopped yellow onions

½ teaspoon kosher salt

¼ teaspoon freshly ground black pepper

½ cup white wine

1 (14-ounce) can fire-roasted diced tomatoes

1 tablespoon tomato paste

1⅓ cups chicken stock

1 bay leaf

1 (15-ounce) can cannellini beans, drained and rinsed

½ cup split red lentils

2 links chicken sausage, halved

4 cloves garlic, smashed with the side of a knife

1 teaspoon sherry vinegar

2 tablespoons chopped fresh flat-leaf parsley or cilantro, plus more for garnish

Bread, for serving

1. In a Dutch oven or other large heavy pot, brown the bacon over medium heat. Scoop out the bacon with a slotted spoon and set aside. Add the breadcrumbs to the pot and stir until they are toasted and golden brown and have absorbed the flavor from the bacon fat. Scoop out the toasted breadcrumbs and set aside.

2. Lower the heat to medium-low and pour in the olive oil. When hot, add the carrots, celery, and onions and cook until the onions are wilted, about 3 minutes. Season with the salt and pepper. Stir in the wine and cook until the liquid is reduced by half, scraping the bottom of the pot with a wooden spoon.

3. Stir in the fire-roasted tomatoes, tomato paste, chicken stock, and bay leaf. Add the beans, lentils, sausage, and garlic. Bring to a boil, then lower the heat to a simmer. Cover the pot and cook, stirring occasionally, until the carrots are tender, about 30 minutes.

4. Stir in the vinegar, reserved bacon, ½ cup of the toasted breadcrumbs, and the parsley. Season to taste with salt and pepper.

5. Serve hot with fresh bread, garnished with the remaining breadcrumbs, herbs, and a drizzle of olive oil, if you wish.

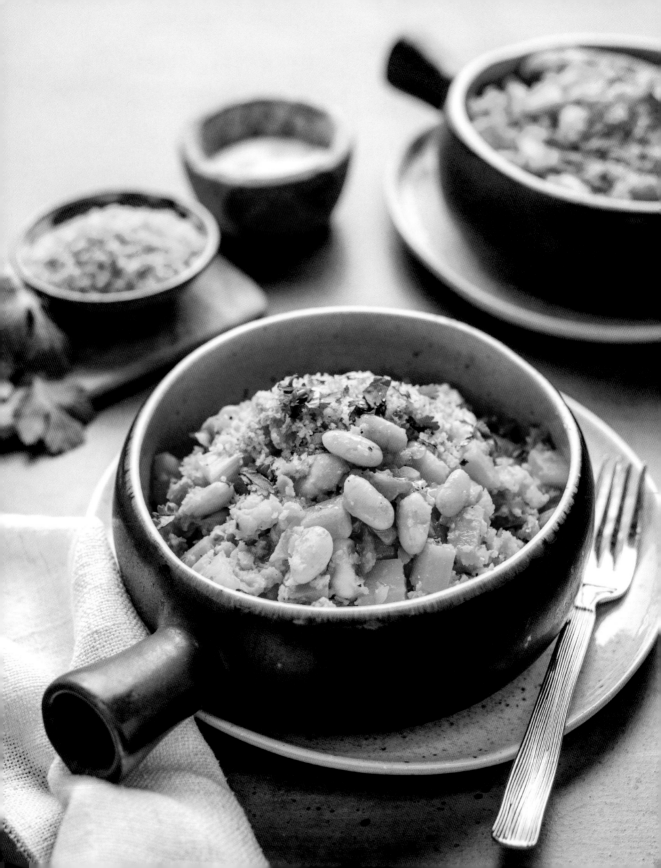

Harissa Chicken Skillet *with* Collard Greens

Yield: 4 servings

Prep Time: 10 minutes, plus 1 hour to marinate chicken

Cook Time: 25 minutes

A bottle of harissa means so many possibilities. It gives the perfect amount of heat in this marinated chicken skillet, served up with vibrant collard greens and roasted red peppers. Feel free to use whichever greens you have on hand for this dish. Try serving it with a side of Corn Tabbouleh (page 132)!

2 tablespoons harissa

1 tablespoon honey

1 tablespoon soy sauce

3 tablespoons extra-virgin olive oil, divided

3 teaspoons minced garlic (3 to 4 cloves), divided

4 boneless, skinless chicken thighs

1 bunch collards, cut into ribbons

1 lemon, halved (optional)

¼ cup sliced roasted red peppers

Chopped fresh cilantro, for garnish

1. In a medium bowl, whisk together the harissa, honey, soy sauce, 1 tablespoon of the olive oil, and 1½ teaspoons of the garlic. Add the chicken and turn to fully coat on all sides with the marinade. Cover the bowl with plastic wrap and refrigerate for at least 1 hour or overnight.

2. When you're ready to cook the chicken, heat the remaining 2 tablespoons of oil in a large skillet over medium heat. When the oil is shimmering, add the chicken and cook for 10 to 15 minutes, turning periodically, until it reaches an internal temperature of 165°F. Transfer the chicken to a plate to rest.

3. Add the collards and lemon, if using, to the skillet and cook for 3 minutes, or until the greens begin to wilt and the lemon is lightly browned. Stir in the remaining 1½ teaspoons of garlic and the roasted red peppers. Return the chicken and any juices to the pan and cook for another 3 minutes. Top with cilantro before serving.

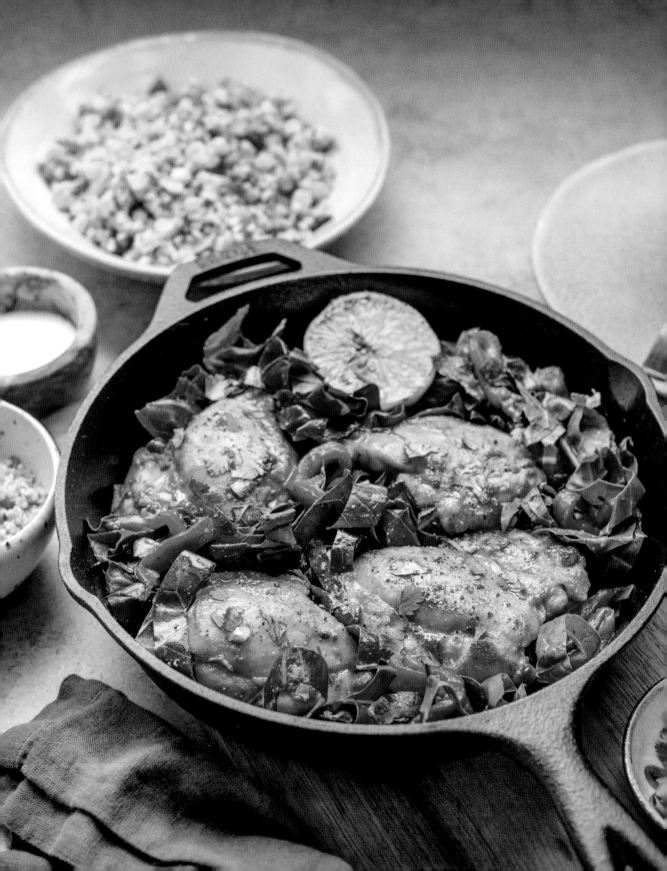

Moroccan-Style Chickpea Stew

Yield: 4 servings
Prep Time: 10 minutes
Cook Time: 40 minutes

When I need something simple but satisfying, I love this chickpea stew simmered in tomatoes and Moroccan spices. If you've never used cinnamon in a savory dish, this is a great place to start—it adds a beautiful warmth to this stew. Combined with a touch of sweetness from golden raisins, it makes for a delicious pantry meal that is perfect for a busy weeknight. It is ideally served with msemen, a Moroccan bread, but if you can't find any, store-bought naan serves just as well!

2 tablespoons extra-virgin olive oil

1 medium yellow onion, diced

2 cloves garlic, minced

2 medium sweet potatoes, peeled and diced

2 teaspoons ground coriander

2 teaspoons ground cumin

1 teaspoon ground cinnamon

1 teaspoon paprika

½ teaspoon cayenne pepper

Kosher salt

1 (14-ounce) can diced tomatoes

1 tablespoon tomato paste

1 teaspoon granulated sugar

1 teaspoon chicken bouillon paste

2 (14-ounce) cans chickpeas, drained and rinsed

2 handfuls chopped kale

¼ cup golden raisins

¼ cup chopped fresh cilantro

Msemen bread or naan, for serving

1. Heat the olive oil in a sauté pan over medium-low heat. Add the onion and garlic and cook until the onion is soft and translucent, about 5 minutes.

2. Stir in the sweet potatoes, coriander, cumin, cinnamon, paprika, cayenne pepper, and a pinch of salt. Cook for about 2 minutes to give the spices time to become fragrant.

3. Stir in the diced tomatoes, tomato paste, sugar, bouillon paste, and chickpeas. Bring to a boil, then lower the heat to a simmer. Cover and simmer for 15 minutes.

4. Uncover the pan. Stir in the kale and raisins and continue simmering, uncovered, for 10 minutes, or until the kale has wilted and the stew has reduced slightly.

5. Garnish with the cilantro and serve immediately with bread.

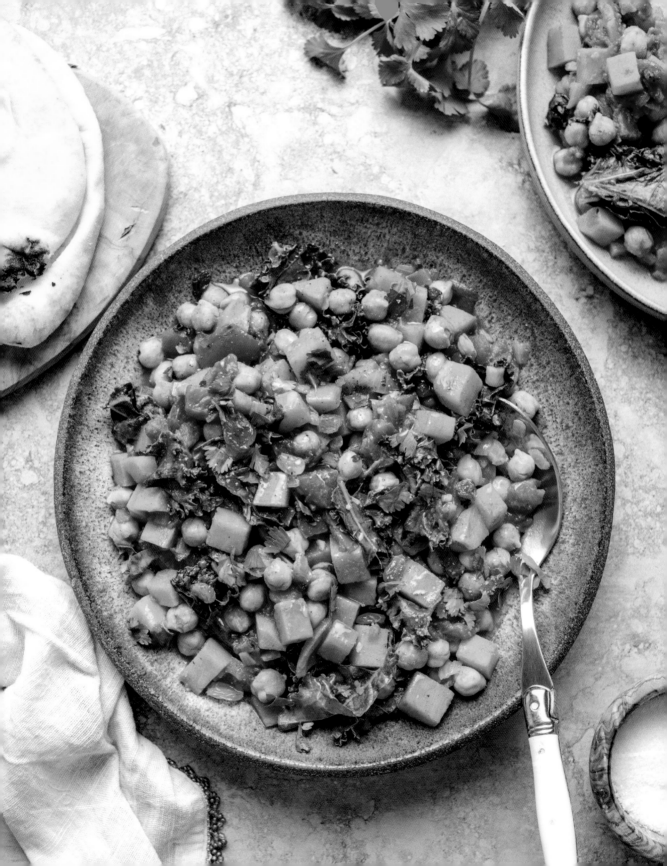

Chicken, Mushroom, *and* Corn Tetrazzini

Yield: 6 to 8 servings
Prep Time: 15 minutes
Cook Time: 45 minutes

I may be in the minority, but I love leftovers! Especially if it means reimagining them into a whole new meal. This casserole is perfect for that leftover rotisserie chicken you bought the other night, Sunday's roast chicken dinner, or the weekend's grilling!

2 tablespoons extra-virgin olive oil

½ cup diced yellow onions (about ½ medium onion)

1 tablespoon minced garlic (3 to 4 cloves)

1 pound cremini or white mushrooms, sliced

1½ cups corn kernels (from about 2 ears)

½ cup green peas

1 teaspoon dried thyme leaves

2 bay leaves

Kosher salt and freshly ground black pepper

¼ cup (½ stick) unsalted butter, plus more for the pan

¼ cup all-purpose flour

2 cup chicken stock, warmed

1 cup whole milk

3 to 4 cups shredded cooked chicken

1 pound linguine, cooked according to package directions

½ cup panko breadcrumbs

½ cup grated Parmigiano-Reggiano cheese

1. Preheat the oven to 350°F with a rack placed in the center of the oven. Lightly butter a 9 by 13-inch (or 2¼-quart) baking dish and set aside.

2. Heat the olive oil in a sauté pan or large skillet over medium-low heat. Add the onions and garlic and cook until the onions are translucent, 3 to 4 minutes. Add the mushrooms, corn, peas, thyme, and bay leaves and season with a pinch each of salt and pepper. Cook until the mushrooms are cooked down and wilted, another 5 minutes. Transfer the mixture to a bowl and set aside.

3. Add the butter to the pan and let it melt. When melted, slowly add the flour, whisking constantly. When the mixture is smooth, whisk in the warm chicken stock and let it simmer, whisking constantly, until the sauce is thick and smooth. Whisk in the milk. Stir in the vegetables and shredded chicken and gently add the cooked noodles. Season with salt and pepper to taste, keeping in mind that the Parmigiano-Reggiano cheese in the topping will add a touch of salt.

4. Transfer the mixture to the buttered baking dish and spread it evenly. Sprinkle with the breadcrumbs and cheese.

5. Bake for about 25 minutes, until the casserole is bubbling and the top is golden brown.

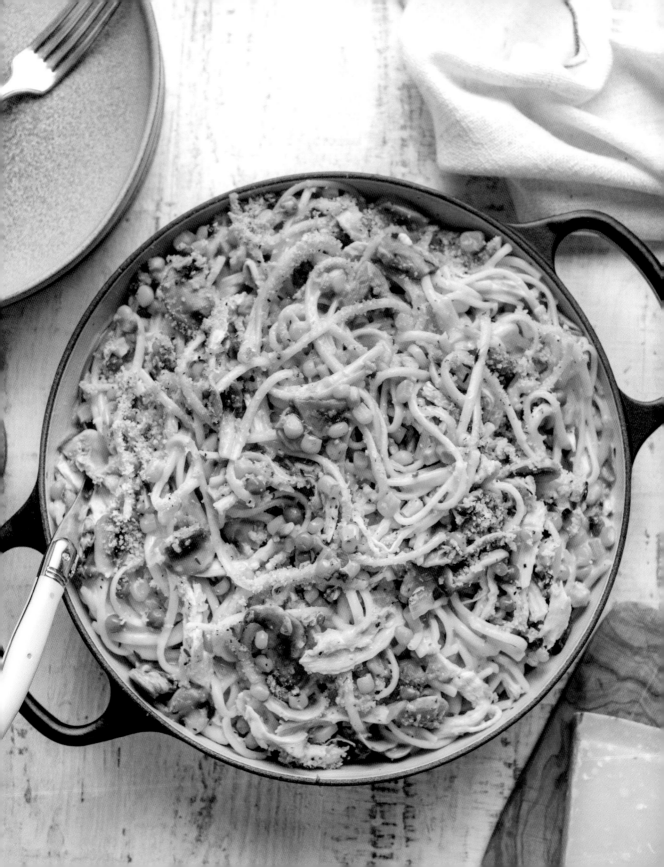

Yield: 4 to 6 servings
Prep Time: 10 minutes
Cook Time: 55 minutes

Vegetable Pot Pie

One of my earliest food memories is of a pot pie that my father ordered when we were on a road trip in Amish country in Pennsylvania. We were eating at a quaint family restaurant that felt more like visiting Grandma's home than a roadside eatery catering to tourists, and I remember my dad tucking into the hot pastry with happiness, revealing the goodness within. It was his kind of food, and I found that it was my kind of food, too. This vegetable pot pie is my simple version of comfort.

¼ cup (½ stick) unsalted butter

½ cup diced yellow onions (about ½ medium onion)

8 ounces cremini or white mushrooms, sliced

1 cup chopped carrots (about 3 medium carrots)

1 cup diced potatoes

½ cup diced sweet potatoes

½ cup green peas

¾ teaspoon kosher salt

Pinch of freshly ground black pepper

¼ cup all-purpose flour

2 cups vegetable stock

½ cup whole milk

¼ teaspoon herbes de Provence

1 sheet puff pastry or pie dough, thawed if frozen

1 large egg beaten with 1 tablespoon whole milk

1. Preheat the oven to 400°F with a rack placed in the center of the oven.

2. Melt the butter in a large heavy skillet over medium-low heat. Add the onions and cook until translucent, about 4 minutes. Increase the heat to medium-high, add the mushrooms, and sauté until the mushrooms have softened, about 2 minutes. Add the carrots, potatoes, sweet potatoes, and peas and stir to combine. Season with the salt and pepper.

3. Sprinkle the flour on top of the vegetables, give them a stir, and cook for a couple of minutes. When the flour starts to bubble, whisk to create a roux. Whisk continuously for about 2 minutes to give the flour a little time to cook.

4. Stir in the vegetable stock, milk, and herbes de Provence. Continue stirring until the gravy is smooth, thick, and bubbling. Lower the heat to a simmer and cook just until the potatoes are fork-tender, another 7 to 8 minutes; be careful not to overcook. Adjust the seasoning to taste with salt and pepper.

5. Transfer the vegetable mixture to a 9-inch round baking dish and let cool to room temperature.

6. Top the baking dish with the puff pastry or pie dough; if you wish, you can cut the pastry or dough into 3-inch rounds and create a pattern over the dish. Brush with the egg wash and bake for 30 to 35 minutes, or until the pastry is golden brown and the filling is hot and bubbly.

7. Serve immediately and enjoy!

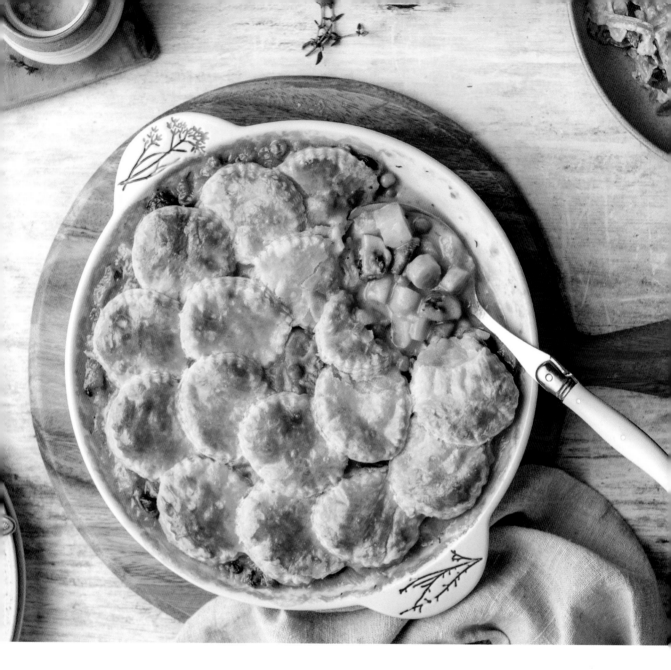

Skirt Steak *with* Peppers, Onions, *and* Barley

Yield: 4 servings

Prep Time: 10 minutes

Cook Time: 35 minutes

Skirt steak is such a flavorful cut of meat, and when sliced and quickly cooked in a heavy skillet with peppers, onions, and hearty pearl barley, it makes for a simple one-pan meal! You don't need a lot of meat in this dish since it's loaded with veggies and fiber-rich barley.

2½ cups beef stock, divided

½ cup pearl barley

8 ounces skirt steak, cut across the grain into 3-inch-long by ¼-inch-wide slices

Kosher salt and freshly ground black pepper

2 teaspoons extra-virgin olive oil

½ lemon (optional)

3 bell peppers, any color, sliced

1 yellow onion, thinly sliced

5 cloves garlic, minced

1 tablespoon tomato paste

1 teaspoon herbes de Provence

½ teaspoon red pepper flakes

Chopped fresh cilantro or basil, for garnish

1. Bring 2 cups of the stock to a boil in a small saucepan over high heat. Add the barley and return to a boil, then reduce the heat to medium and cover the pan. Cook according to the package directions, usually 20 to 30 minutes. When done, drain any excess broth and set aside. Meanwhile, cook the steak and vegetables.

2. Generously season the steak slices on all sides with salt and pepper. Heat the olive oil in a large heavy skillet over high heat. Sear the steak for 1 to 5 minutes per side, working in batches if necessary. Transfer the steak to a plate.

3. If using the lemon, sear it cut side down in the skillet until it has softened, about 2 minutes. Remove from the pan and set aside.

4. Lower the heat to medium. Add the bell peppers, onion, and garlic and season with 1 teaspoon of salt and a pinch of pepper. Cook, stirring occasionally, until the onions have wilted, 4 to 5 minutes.

5. Stir in the remaining ½ cup of stock, the tomato paste, herbes de Provence, and red pepper flakes and bring to a simmer. Stir in the cooked barley and reserved steak, allowing the beef and barley to reheat. Garnish with the charred lemon half and cilantro and serve immediately.

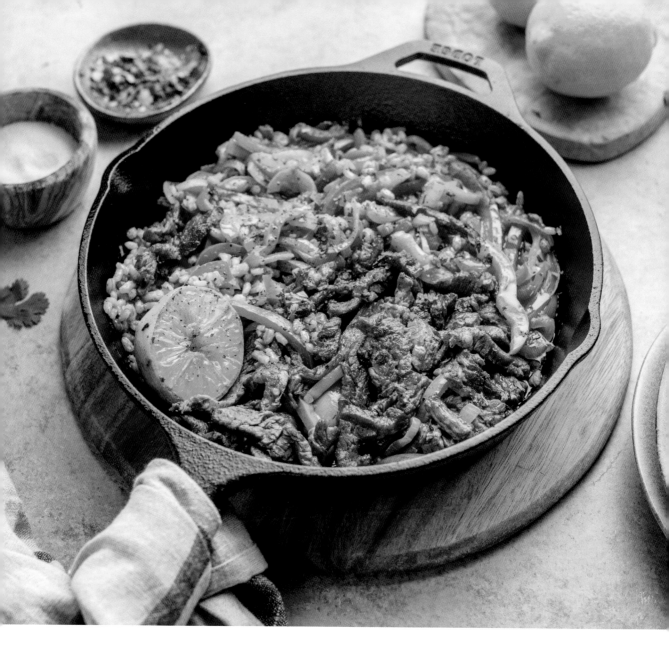

NOTE

Quick-cooking pearl barley has had its outer husk and bran removed and is easily found in markets. Hulled barley is the whole-grain variety and definitely more wholesome; however, it takes more time to cook. Use whichever you have on hand; if you use hulled barley, add another 5 to 7 minutes of cooking time.

Butternut Squash Butter Chicken

Yield: 4 servings

Prep Time: 15 minutes, plus 30 minutes to marinate chicken

Cook Time: 30 minutes

My first job after college landed me in perhaps the best location I could have hoped for: midtown Manhattan. My office was within walking distance of many delicious restaurants. A block away, my favorite Indian restaurant served up an irresistible butter chicken, which I craved long after I moved out of New York. When I decided to tackle butter chicken at home, I found I could still get the flavors I craved while lightening up the dish with a butternut squash puree. My son is a huge fan of this meal, and for years he had no idea that he was mopping up servings of butternut squash with his naan (although the secret's out now!).

FOR THE MARINATED CHICKEN:

½ cup plain whole milk yogurt

1 tablespoon fresh lemon juice

1 tablespoon grated fresh ginger

1½ teaspoons minced garlic (about 2 cloves)

2 teaspoons garam masala

1 teaspoon ground cumin

1 teaspoon turmeric powder

½ teaspoon chili powder

½ teaspoon kosher salt

1 pound chicken tenders, cut into 2-inch pieces

1½ tablespoons ghee or unsalted butter, for the pan

FOR THE BUTTER SAUCE:

1½ tablespoons ghee or unsalted butter, divided

½ cup chopped yellow onions

2 cloves garlic, minced

1 teaspoon grated fresh ginger

½ teaspoon chili powder

½ teaspoon garam masala

½ teaspoon ground cumin

1 cup diced butternut squash

1 cup canned crushed tomatoes

¼ cup water

¼ cup heavy cream

1½ teaspoons granulated sugar

1 teaspoon kosher salt

Pinch of cayenne pepper (optional)

FOR SERVING/GARNISH:

Cooked white basmati rice

Fresh cilantro

Toasted naan

1. In a medium bowl, whisk together the yogurt, lemon juice, ginger, garlic, spices, and salt. Add the chicken and stir to coat. Cover the bowl with plastic wrap and refrigerate for at least 30 minutes or overnight—the longer the chicken marinates, the better!

2. When you're ready to cook the chicken, heat the ghee in a sauté pan over medium-high heat. Remove the chicken from the marinade; discard the marinade. Add the chicken to the pan and cook for about 3 minutes; it will not be fully cooked at this point. Transfer the chicken to a plate and set aside.

3. Make the sauce: Heat the ghee in the same sauté pan over medium heat. Add the onions, garlic, and ginger and cook for 5 minutes, or until the onions begin to wilt. Stir in the spices, butternut squash, tomatoes, and water. Lower the heat to a simmer and let the sauce bubble for 10 minutes, or until the squash is fork-tender. Remove from

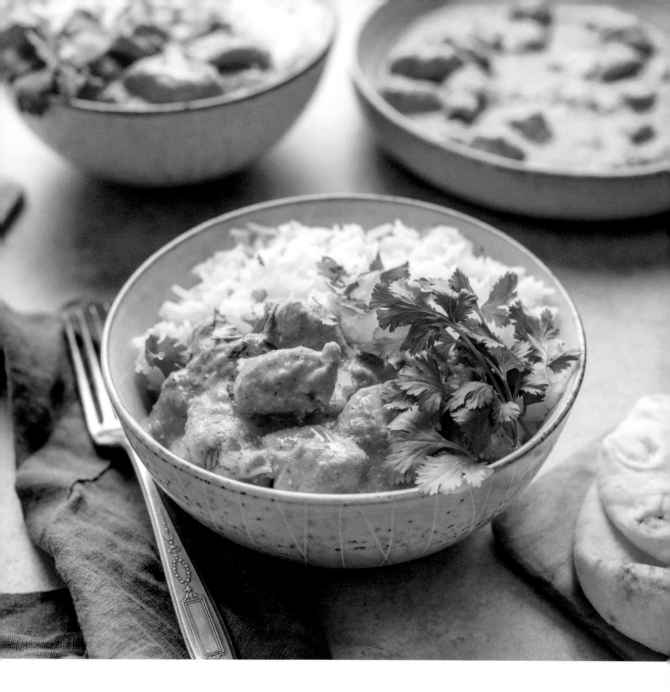

the heat, transfer to a blender, and purée until smooth, working in batches if necessary.

4. Pour the sauce back into the pan, add the chicken, and stir in the cream, sugar, salt, and cayenne, if using. Simmer for another 10 minutes, or until the chicken is fully cooked.

5. Spoon the chicken over rice, garnish with cilantro, and serve with toasted naan on the side.

Yield: 4 servings

Prep Time: 15 minutes, plus 30 minutes to marinate pork

Cook Time: 10 minutes

Grilled Pork *and* Vegetable Skewers

One of my favorite things about living in California is that we can grill nearly year-round, and grilling is, perhaps, my favorite kind of cooking. A simple marinade can do wonders, and grilled veggies are irresistible! These skewers are pretty much a meal on a stick, but I like to make sure there are extra veggies to serve alongside. Since the meat and veggies are cut into bite-sized pieces, the skewers cook in just about 10 minutes.

4 cloves garlic, minced

2 tablespoons balsamic vinegar

1 teaspoon Dijon mustard

2 teaspoons kosher salt

½ teaspoon freshly ground black pepper

3 tablespoons extra-virgin olive oil, divided

1 pork tenderloin (about 1 pound), cut into 1-inch cubes

1 small red onion

2 yellow squash

2 zucchini

SPECIAL EQUIPMENT:

6 to 8 (9-inch) wooden or stainless-steel skewers

1. In a glass (or nonreactive) bowl, whisk together the garlic, vinegar, mustard, salt, pepper, and 2 tablespoons of the olive oil. Add the pork, stirring well to coat the meat on all sides with the marinade. Cover the bowl with plastic wrap and refrigerate for at least 30 minutes or overnight.

2. If using wooden skewers, soak them in water for 30 minutes before grilling to prevent them from burning.

3. Preheat a grill to medium-high heat.

4. Peel the red onion and slice it in half lengthwise. Cut into wedges about 1½ inches in size. Slice the yellow squash and zucchini into 1-inch rounds. Place all the vegetables in a bowl, drizzle with the remaining tablespoon of olive oil, season generously with salt and pepper, and toss to evenly coat.

5. Thread the pork, red onion, yellow squash, and zucchini onto the skewers. If you have extra vegetables (and you likely will), grill them either skewered or in a grill basket.

6. Grill the skewers for about 10 minutes, rotating once or twice, until fully cooked; the meat should have an internal temperature of 145°F.

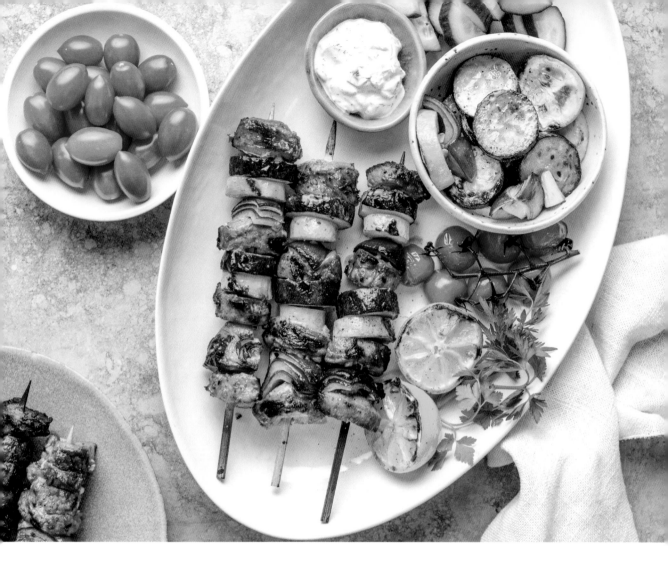

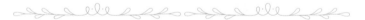

NOTES

The pork can be prepped and marinated the night before—the longer it sits in the marinade, the better!

If using metal skewers, you can also thread the ingredients onto the skewers the night before. If you opt for wooden skewers, I recommend skewering right before grilling to ensure that the wood still has moisture from soaking to prevent the skewers from burning.

These skewers are delicious served on their own, but they're also wonderful with tzatziki (page 76). It adds a nice zing to the meat and veggies and makes for a simple and satisfying meal.

Acknowledgments

Once you write a book, the acknowledgments page transforms from an overlooked and often-skipped page to perhaps the single most meaningful leaf in the entire book. Looking back after all these months of writing, testing, and photographing, I know I could not have done it without the support of others.

Firstly, to my husband, Thomas, thank you for your patience as I fully immersed myself in creating this cookbook. I was constantly in the kitchen, behind a computer screen, wrangling food and cameras on set, filling the refrigerator and freezer to the brim with food you were not allowed to touch, and burning the midnight oil, even on weekends. You dealt with my stress, picked up ingredients, were woefully ignored, and still, you encouraged me every step of the way. I could not have done this without you.

To my children, Caeli and Carsten, thank you for eating your veggies, for taste testing, and for also understanding my constant push to work. I hope that one day, you'll cook from this book and remember this year with good memories. I love you both. You are the reason I do everything I do.

To Holly Jennings, for your eagle eye and awe-inspiring wordsmithing, for making my words match my thoughts, and for molding the manuscript into something even better than I could have hoped. I am so grateful!

To Pam Mourouzis, Stephanie Lippitt, Susan Lloyd, Lance Freimuth, and everyone at Victory Belt, for welcoming me, believing in me, and making this process so incredibly rewarding.

To Ellen Finstad, Helena Bohdanovych, and Vladi Vasylenkov, for your thoughtful work behind the scenes. I couldn't run my business without you, most especially while I worked on this project.

To my sister, Lianne, who in your darkest days would encourage me when it should have been I encouraging you. I love you. And to Niall, for loving Lianne (and us all).

To my brother, Andre, who holds down the fort on the East Coast. I appreciate all you do, especially when I struggle being so far away. Thank you to you and Jamie so, so much.

To Dad, who taught me the value of hard work, corned beef, and "in onion there is strength." The corned beef in this book is for you and for all those nights when Mom was at work.

To Mom, whose presence I feel every day. Thank you for teaching me to love life, good food, and travel. I miss you so very much.

To Tita Leah, for teaching me to cook and to nourish others.

To Mom Baker, I am so blessed to have you in my life. Thank you for loving me dearly.

To Aysegul Sanford and Traci York, for our monthly chats. You are the best cheerleaders and "coworkers" I could ask for.

To Toni Dash, for always being just a phone call away.

To Amar Yadav, Amy To, and Karen Ho—it takes a village, and I appreciate the Squams so much. Our lunches helped with my sanity through this process! Thank you all for your friendship.

And last but not least, thank you to my readers at Kitchen Confidante. Thank you for cooking with me—it is because of you that I get to do what I love most, every single day of my life.

Recipe Index

Breakfasts

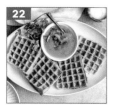
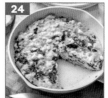
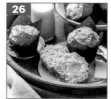
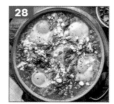
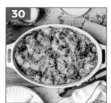
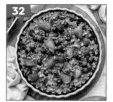
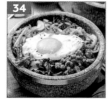
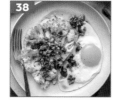
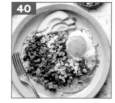
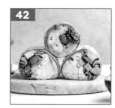
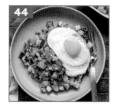

Appetizers and Small Plates

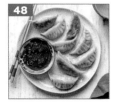

Jackfruit Dumplings
(Gyoza)

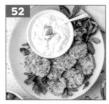

Zucchini Fritters

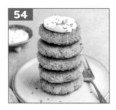

Sweet Potato
Patties

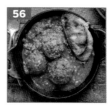

Mushroom
Meatballs

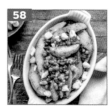

Pork and Beans
Poutine

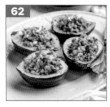

Stuffed Acorn
Squash with Farro,
Kale, and White
Beans

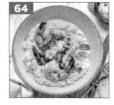

Shrimp and
Cauliflower Grits

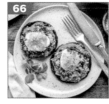

Stuffed Portobello
Mushrooms and
Spicy Romesco
Sauce

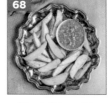

Steak Fries with
Chimichurri

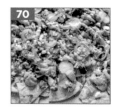

Veggie Nachos

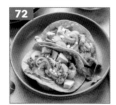

Spicy Cauliflower
Tacos

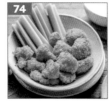

Buffalo Cauliflower
"Wings"

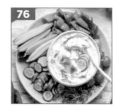

Tzatziki

Sandwiches, Flatbreads, and Burgers

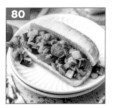
80 Ratatouille Sandwiches with Chicken Sausage

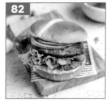
82 Mushroom Burgers

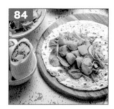
84 Spiced Potato Wraps

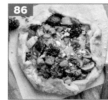
86 Roasted Vegetable Galette

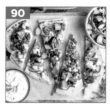
90 Gyro Flatbread with Cucumber Salad

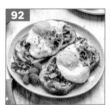
92 Avocado Toast with Eggs and Bacon

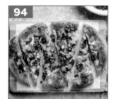
94 Roasted Winter Squash, Kale, and Turkey Bacon Pizza

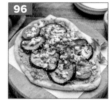
96 Roasted Eggplant Flatbread

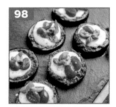
98 Mini Eggplant Pizzas

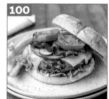
100 Veggie Bacon Burgers

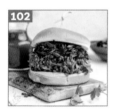
102 Lentil Pulled Pork Sandwiches

Soups

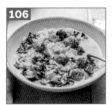
106 Italian Wedding Soup

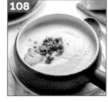
108 Creamy Cauliflower Soup with Pancetta

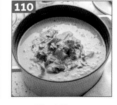
110 Thai Curry Butternut Squash Lentil Soup

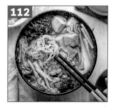
112 Veggie Miso Ramen

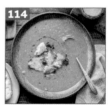
114 Roasted Tomato Soup au Pistou

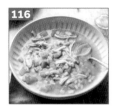

116

Chicken Corn Soup

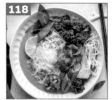

118

Thai-Style Chicken Noodle Vegetable Soup

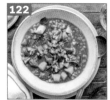

120

Roasted Tomatillo Tortilla Soup

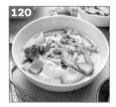

122

Vegetable, Beef, and Barley Soup

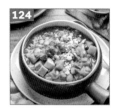

124

Kabocha Squash Chili

Salads

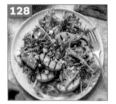

128

Grilled Peach Salad with Goat Cheese

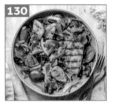

130

Grilled Fig and Halloumi Salad

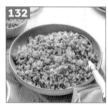

132

Corn Tabbouleh

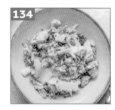

134

Brussels Sprouts Caesar Salad

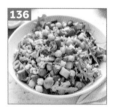

136

Chickpea Summer Salad

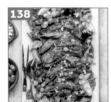

138

Flank Steak and Artichoke Salad

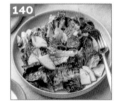

140

Little Gem Salad with Apple and Beets

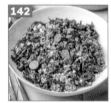

142

Kale Quinoa Salad with Grapes

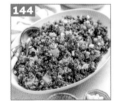

144

Winter Squash Quinoa Salad

Bowls

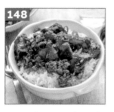
148
Eggplant and Pork Bowls with Black Bean Sauce

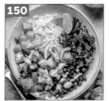
150
Roasted Sweet Potato and Chipotle Black Bean Bowls

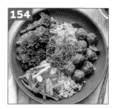
154
Adobo Meatball Bowls

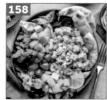
158
Curry Chicken Salad Bowls

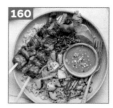
160
Beef Satay Bowls with Cucumber and Carrot Slaw

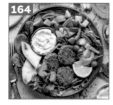
164
Falafel Bowls

Pasta and Noodles

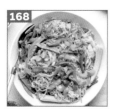
168
Stir-Fried Vegetable Chow Mein

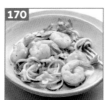
170
Coconut Zucchini Noodles with Shrimp

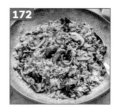
172
Brown Butter Orzo with Mushrooms and Kale

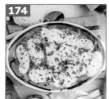
174
Eggplant Lasagna

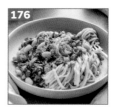
176
Linguine with Beans and Swiss Chard

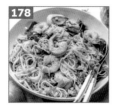
178
Pasta with Spicy Shrimp and Corn

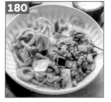
180
Garlicky Sweet Potato Noodles with Vegetable Ragu

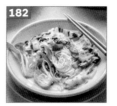
182
Somen Noodles in a Creamy Coconut Broth with Bok Choy

Hearty Plates

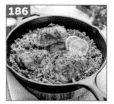
186 Broccoli Rice Chicken Skillet

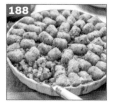
188 Turkey Tater Tot Casserole

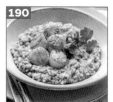
190 Spinach Risotto with Scallops

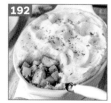
192 Winter Vegetable Shepherd's Pie

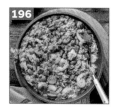
196 Jambalaya Skillet

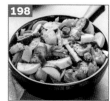
198 Filipino Pinakbet (Vegetable Pork Stew)

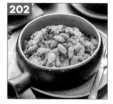
202 Vegetable Cassoulet

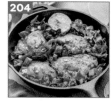
204 Harissa Chicken Skillet with Collard Greens

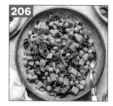
206 Moroccan-Style Chickpea Stew

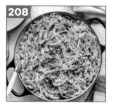
208 Chicken, Mushroom, and Corn Tetrazzini

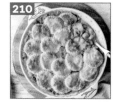
210 Vegetable Pot Pie

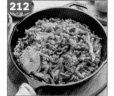
212 Skirt Steak with Peppers, Onions, and Barley

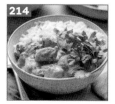
214 Butternut Squash Butter Chicken

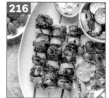
216 Grilled Pork and Vegetable Skewers

General Index

D–E

F